Muna Beesi, M.D.
00615

ASSISTED VENTILATION

ASSISTED VENTILATION

SECOND EDITION

Edited by

John Moxham, MD, FRCP
Professor of Thoracic Medicine,
King's College School of Medicine
and Dentistry, London

and

John Goldstone, MD, FRCA
Senior Lecturer in Anaesthesia
University College London Medical School

BMJ
Publishing
Group

© BMJ Publishing Group 1991, 1994

First published in 1991
Second edition 1994
by the BMJ Publishing Group, BMA House, Tavistock Square,
London WC1H 9JR

British Library Cataloguing in Publication Data

A catalogue record for this book is available
from the British Library

ISBN 0-7279-0843-X

With acknowledgement to *Thorax*, in which the chapters in this book were originally
published.

Typeset, printed and bound in Great Britain by
Latimer Trend & Company Ltd, Plymouth

Contents

Introduction

JOHN MOXHAM, JOHN GOLDSTONE

This book consists of contributions from thoracic physicians, intensive care specialists, and anaesthetists. Its purpose is to provide comprehensive, up-to-date information about assisted ventilation aimed at thoracic and general physicians, as well as critical care physicians, and anaesthetists in training. It is our view that it is helpful for all staff caring for patients on the intensive care unit to be familiar with assisted ventilation techniques.

Chapter 1 describes the techniques of assisted ventilation that are available on the intensive care unit and seeks to unravel the jargon and explain the equipment. Too frequently, physicians and other medical staff on the unit do not know the details of ventilation technique. Chapter 2 deals with the indications for assisted ventilation; it is as important to appreciate the limitations of the technique as much as its possibilities. We hope this section will contribute to the debate that so frequently occurs between physician and anaesthetist about the merits of ventilating particular patients.

Ventilated patients are totally dependent on those caring for them. Thus to care for the intubated patient is a complex and demanding task. Chapter 3 seeks to discuss the many and varied aspects of the general care of intubated patients.

For most ventilated patients on the intensive care unit the withdrawal of assisted ventilation is straightforward, but in a minority weaning presents great difficulties. These difficulties often cause concern and frustration. Chapter 4 seeks to explain why some patients fail to wean, what can be done to facilitate the weaning process, and so to demystify this complex clinical situation.

For most patients assisted ventilation occurs on the intensive care unit, but, increasingly, selected patients are receiving ventilation within the community, most commonly to control the nocturnal hypoventilation associated with skeletal and neuromuscular diseases such as kyphoscoliosis. Non-invasive ventilation techniques have had a substantial clinical impact and the indications for domiciliary ventilation, and hospital based ventilation outside the intensive care unit, have substantially broadened. Chapter 5 discusses this important area of non-invasive ventilation. It is now appropriate for thoracic physicians, including those in training, as well as critical care specialists and anaesthetists, to be fully familiar with non-invasive ventilatory techniques. It is very likely that this clinical arena will continue to expand.

We hope that the reader, having worked through the indications for ventilation, the techniques available, the general care of intubated patients, the problems of weaning, and the question of non-invasive ventilation, will feel that there is not too much in the field of assisted ventilation that is likely to cause him or her anxiety.

We trust that this short and practical account of assisted ventilation will be of value to all those who read it. We would certainly welcome any suggestions for improvement of future editions.

1 Artificial ventilation: history, equipment, and techniques

J D YOUNG, M K SYKES

Brief history of artificial ventilators

An artificial ventilator is essentially a device that replaces or augments the function of the inspiratory muscles, providing the necessary energy to ensure an adequate flow of gas into the alveoli during inspiration. When this support is removed, gas is expelled as the lung and chest wall recoil to their original volume; exhalation is a passive process. In the earliest reports of artificial ventilation this energy was provided by the respiratory muscles of another person, as expired air resuscitation. Baker[1] has traced references to expired air resuscitation in the newborn as far back as 1472, and in adults there is a report of an asphyxiated miner being revived with mouth-to-mouth resuscitation in 1744. In the eighteenth century, artificial ventilation using bellows became the accepted first line treatment for drowning victims.[2] Automatic artificial ventilators which did not require a human power source took another 150 years to appear, and were first suggested by Fell[3] and then made available commercially by Draeger[4] in 1907. These were still devices for resuscitation, for the Draeger company, at that time, was noted for its mine rescue apparatus.

The major stimulus for the introduction of intermittent positive pressure ventilation was the need to prevent paradoxical respiration and mediastinal shift when surgeons carried out chest surgery. By 1940, Crafoord[5] was able to report the successful use of the "Spiropulsator" in over 100 patients undergoing thoracic surgery. A further boost to the development of automatic artificial ventilators occurred in 1952, when a catastrophic poliomyelitis epidemic struck Denmark. There was a very high incidence of bulbar in-

1

volvement and of 866 patients with paralysis admitted over a period of 19 weeks, 316 required postural drainage, tracheostomy, or respiratory support. By using tracheostomy and manual positive pressure ventilation the Danish physicians reduced the mortality from poliomyelitis from 80% at the beginning of the epidemic to 40% at the end. The artificial ventilation was carried out entirely by hand; 1400 university students worked in shifts to keep the patients ventilated. The fear that another epidemic might afflict Europe expedited research into powered mechanical ventilators.

Classification of artificial ventilators

The lungs can be artificially ventilated either by reducing the ambient pressure around the thorax (negative pressure ventilation) or by increasing the pressure within the airways (positive pressure ventilation). Negative pressure ventilators use a rigid chamber that encloses either the thorax (cuirass) or the whole body below the neck (tank respirator or "iron lung"). The pressure in the chamber is cyclically reduced using a large volume displacement pump; this causes the lungs to expand and contract. Such ventilators were used extensively for poliomyelitis victims, and are still in use today for long term respiratory support or overnight support for patients with respiratory muscle weakness. Tank ventilators, however, occupy a great deal of space and access to the patient is poor, so they are not suitable for use in general intensive care units. There has been a recent revival of interest in negative pressure ventilators in paediatric intensive care units to avoid the need for endotracheal intubation,[6] and a cuirass system capable of ventilating at normal and high frequencies is now marketed (the "Hayek oscillator").

There are several systems for classifying the functional characteristics of positive pressure artificial ventilators,[7] but most of these predate the introduction of the modern, servo-controlled ventilators. The classification system that has been adopted by the International and British Standards Organizations is that of Mapleson.[8] This classification is based on two ventilator characteristics: the method by which gas is driven into the patient during inspiration and the way the machine cycles between inspiration and expiration. The first characteristic divides all machines into flow generators and pressure generators. A flow generator produces a predetermined pattern of gas flow during inspiration, and this pattern is little affected by changes in respiratory compliance or

2

resistance. A pressure generator produces a preset pattern of pressure in the airway and since this is relatively low, the rate of lung inflation depends not only on the pressure, but also on the respiratory resistance and compliance that determine the time constant of the respiratory system.

In general, a flow generator ventilator is used for adults, and a pressure generator ventilator for children, though the latter may be used in adults when control of peak airway pressure is important. The pressure generator is particularly useful in children where uncuffed endotracheal tubes are used and there is a leak of gas around the endotracheal tube during inspiration. A pressure generator tends to compensate for this leak by increasing the flow into the airway, whereas a proportion of the tidal volume is lost with a flow generator.

The second property of the ventilator is the mechanism which causes it to cycle between inspiration and expiration. Ventilators that switch between inspiration and expiration after a preset time interval are termed time cycled, those that switch when a preset airway pressure threshold has been reached are termed pressure cycled and those that cycle when a preset tidal volume has been delivered are termed volume cycled. Cycling from expiration to inspiration is usually effected by a timing mechanism or by a triggering device which senses the subatmospheric pressure or the flow generated in the inspiratory tube by the patient's inspiratory effort.

This traditional classification was devised during a period when ventilators were totally mechanical, and driven either by compressed gas or by an electrically powered piston or bellows. By 1954, however, Donald had used an electronic trigger which initiated inspiration and in 1958 an electronic timing device was incorporated in the Barnet ventilator.[9] In 1971, the Siemens–Elema company introduced the Servo 900 ventilator, which combined a simple pneumatic system with a sophisticated electronic measuring and control unit.[10] Gas flow to and from the patient's lungs was controlled by a pair of scissor valves and monitored with pressure and flow sensors. The control unit adjusted the scissor valves to ensure that the flow patterns measured by the sensors corresponded to those selected by the operator. This method of control is termed a servo or feedback system and is very flexible. Potentially one machine can mimic all the previously described categories of ventilator. Although the Mapleson classification can still be used

3

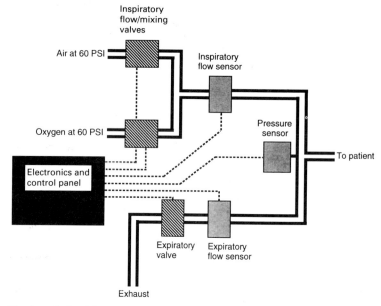

Fɪɢ 1.1—A simplified diagram of a modern intensive care ventilator.

to describe the individual ventilatory modes of modern ventilators, it cannot be used to describe the ventilator itself.

Modern intensive care ventilators

Modern ventilators owe their existence to a combination of advanced microprocessor-based electronics and high speed, electrically actuated, gas control valves. Combining these with pressure and flow sensors allows very sophisticated servo-controlled ventilators to be produced. In the early machines, the inspired gases were premixed and the total flow controlled by an electronically actuated valve. In the most recent machines, both mixing and control of flow are effected by a valve on each gas line. A simplified diagram of a modern ventilator is shown in figure 1.1. Compressed air and oxygen are delivered to two high speed, electrically operated, proportional gas control valves that act as the inspiratory valve controlling both inspiratory flow and oxygen tension. The release of gas from the lungs is controlled by an electrically actuated expiratory valve. All the valves are under the control of an electronic

4

control unit containing one or more microprocessors. The airway pressure and flow of gas into the patient are monitored by the pressure and inspiratory flow sensors. The expiratory flow can also be monitored to check for leaks and disconnection of the patient from the ventilator. This design enables the ventilator to be used as either a flow or a pressure generator. For example, if the operator selects a constant flow during inspiration (intermittent positive pressure ventilation with a constant inspiratory flow rate) the ventilator will open the inspiratory valves until the inspiratory flow sensor measures the required flow. If the inspiratory flow decreases the inspiratory valves will be opened further to compensate, and vice versa. If the operator wishes the ventilator to act as a constant pressure generator (for example in inspiratory pressure support), the ventilator will open the inspiratory valves until the pressure sensor indicates the desired pressure has been reached. The ventilator will then maintain the airway pressure at the desired level by opening or closing the inspiratory valves. Expiration is achieved by closing the inspiratory valves and opening the expiratory valves. The bulk of a modern ventilator is now the electronic unit and the pneumatic units are often very compact.

The use of electronic feedback systems in ventilators has many advantages. The moving parts within the ventilator are kept to a minimum, sophisticated alarm systems are possible, the ventilators can be made physically small, and maintenance and repair are simple. Figure 1.2 shows the control panel of a Puritan–Bennett 7200 series ventilator. All the controls are electronic, there is no mechanical linkage between the controls and the valves. If a new mode of ventilation appears to be useful clinically it can generally be added to an existing machine by altering the software in the electronic unit. We have now reached a situation where our ability to produce new modes of artificial ventilation far exceeds our ability to test them clinically.

Interactions between patients and ventilators

As early as 1929 it was observed that a patient who "fought" the ventilator, struggling to breathe and not synchronising his respiratory efforts with the ventilator, was difficult to manage and suffered complications.[11] To minimise these problems, many ventilated patients were heavily sedated, and in some cases paralysed with neuromuscular blocking agents (for example, pan-

5

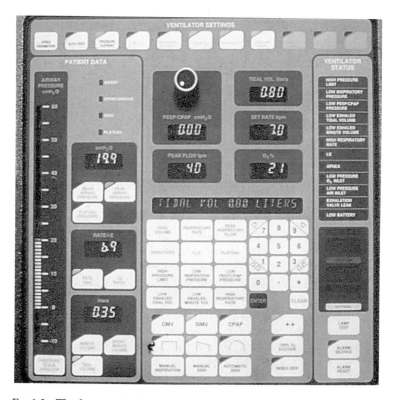

FIG 1.2—The front panel of a Puritan–Bennett 7200 series ventilator. The panel is divided into a control area (centre), a measurement area (left), and an alarm area (right). The controls are all electronic, and extensive use is made of menus, which appear in the display window, to control and set the ventilator. Specialist modes of ventilation, software upgrades, and options are available from the row of buttons at the top of the panel.

curonium). In the early 1980s, paralysis of ventilated patients was very common in British intensive care units,[12][13] and heavy sedation was used to dissociate the patients from their surroundings.

Paralysis of ventilated patients is not without risks.[14] The paralysed patient is unable to make any spontaneous respiratory effort, so a disconnection from the ventilator is rapidly fatal if not detected. There is a risk that the patient may be aware of his or her surroundings but unable to communicate, and the risk of pulmonary embolus is probably increased. Even sedative drugs are not without risk,[15] as shown by the marked increase in the mortality

6

of trauma patients given etomidate infusions that led to suppression of adrenal activity.

Only a few clinicians now favour deep sedation and paralysis,[16] the preferred approach being a comfortable patient who can be aroused easily and can communicate with the staff. To achieve this goal, ventilators have to be more flexible and adapt to the needs of the patient, rather than sedating and paralysing the patient to overcome the inadequacies of the ventilator. In its simplest form this is achieved by inserting a valve into the ventilator tubing that allows the patient to breath spontaneously from another gas source between the breaths delivered by the ventilator. This mode of ventilation is termed intermittent mandatory ventilation (IMV) and was initially used as a technique to wean patients from mechanical ventilation to spontaneous respiration. By 1987, however, over 70% of American intensive care units were using IMV as their primary mode of ventilatory support.[17] IMV is not an interactive mode of ventilation. The ventilator continues to deliver the preset pattern of breaths regardless of the patient's respiratory effort. Therefore, a patient could take a spontaneous breath and then immediately receive a second additional breath from the ventilator, so causing lung overdistension. This is usually referred to as "stacking" of breaths. The newer microprocessor-controlled ventilators not only allow the patient to breathe spontaneously and receive IMV breaths from the ventilator circuit but also incorporate several "smart" modes of ventilation, where the ventilator can sense the patient's respiratory effort by sensing pressure or flow changes in the ventilator tubing and then adjust the ventilatory support accordingly. Not only does this avoid stacking and other problems with ventilator–patient synchronisation, but it also allows graded respiratory assistance with every breath. The most common synchronised methods used are synchronised intermittent mandatory ventilation (SIMV), and inspiratory pressure support (IPS). Examples of the pressure/time waveforms produced by the different modes of ventilation are shown in figure 1.3.

Ventilatory strategies in common use

Intermittent positive pressure ventilation
Each year millions of patients are ventilated during anaesthesia for surgical procedures requiring muscular relaxation. Nearly all of these patients are ventilated with basic intermittent positive pressure

7

ventilation (IPPV), using simple mechanical ventilators. For short periods of respiratory support these ventilators are perfectly adequate, because the patient is both paralysed and anaesthetised there is no need for interactive ventilators. Weaning is accomplished by reversing the muscle relaxation and lightening the anaesthetic. In intensive care units this mode of ventilation is used for patients who have to be heavily sedated and paralysed to treat their primary

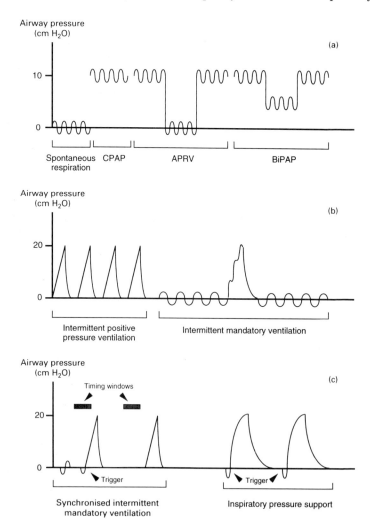

condition (for example, tetanus) or for those who are unable to make any respiratory movement (for example, in those with severe Guillain–Barré syndrome). Intermittent positive pressure ventilation can be undertaken with almost any artificial ventilator, mechanical or servo-controlled, as no special refinements are needed. In the United States, intermittent positive pressure ventilation is usually referred to as controlled mechanical ventilation (CMV).

The essential settings for IPPV are the tidal volume and respiratory rate. Conventional settings are a tidal volume of 10–12 ml/kg and a respiratory rate of 8–10 breaths per minute. The third setting, not usually quoted, is the inspiratory to expiratory time ratio (I:E ratio). In ventilators from European and Scandinavian manufacturers this is usually set by the operator (at 1:2–1:3) and the ventilator then calculates the gas flow rate required during inspiration to achieve the required tidal volume. In ventilators from North America it is more common for the operator to specify the maximum gas flow during inspiration, the machine then calculates the I:E ratio. The gas flow during inspiration can be constant or can follow a number of different patterns (for example, sine or decelerating). No one pattern has been shown to be better than another. As with all modes of ventilation, the inspired oxygen concentration and the mean lung volume (manipulated using the I:E ratio and added positive end expiratory pressure) determine the arterial oxygen tension, and the tidal volume and respiratory rate determine the arterial carbon dioxide tension.

FIG 1.3—The effects of different forms of ventilation on airway pressure. (a) The modes of ventilation that require spontaneous respiration by the patient are shown. CPAP is spontaneous ventilation at an increased mean airway pressure. In APRV and BiPAP the mean airway pressure is altered periodically to increase the minute ventilation and hence carbon dioxide clearance. (b) Shows intermittent positive pressure ventilation and intermittent mandatory ventilation, which is in effect spontaneous respiration with superimposed intermittent positive pressure ventilation. As there is no patient–ventilator interaction during intermittent mandatory ventilation, the patient continues to breathe even during the mandatory breath. (c) Shows synchronised ventilator modes. Synchronised intermittent mandatory ventilation gives mandatory breaths triggered by the patient making an inspiratory effort. If the patient fails to make an inspiratory effort within a preset time period (the timing window) the ventilator will deliver an unsynchronised mandatory breath to maintain minute ventilation. In inspiratory pressure support every respiratory effort causes the ventilator to increase the airway pressure to a preset value and so assist the patient's own inspiratory effort.

Patients who are anaesthetised, comatose, or who have recently undergone abdominal surgery have a reduced functional residual capacity. The reduction can be sufficient to cause airway closure in dependent areas of the lung before the end of expiration, leading to underventilation of these areas and a mismatch of ventilation and perfusion.[18] This in turn leads to hypoxaemia. The functional residual capacity can be maintained by leaving a constant standing pressure on the lungs, keeping them slightly inflated even at the end of expiration; this is positive end expiratory pressure (PEEP). The use of PEEP, and how best to determine its optimum level, has been the subject of debate for many years. On the positive side, PEEP causes an increase in arterial oxygen tension for the same inspired oxygen tension. On the negative side, the constantly raised intrathoracic pressure causes a diminution in venous return to the heart, a decrease in cardiac output and an increased risk of pneumothorax. The controversy may now be resolved, for a recent study showed that mortality increased with the aggressive application of PEEP and that the minimum PEEP which kept arterial oxygenation within acceptable limits was "best PEEP".[19] PEEP may be used with any of the ventilatory methods described here.

Synchronised intermittent positive pressure ventilation
To avoid stacking of breaths during IMV the ventilator must be able to sense that the patient has taken a breath, and then avoid delivering a mandatory (ventilator delivered) breath during the period of the spontaneous breath. This level of sophistication was not easily achieved before electronic control was used in artificial ventilators. One of the first machines to have an SIMV facility was the Servo 900B, a refinement of the original Servo 900. This machine dispensed with external IMV valves and used its internal valves and sensors to provide SIMV. Any spontaneous inspiratory activity by the patient was sensed as a reduction in pressure in the gas circuit by the pressure sensor. The expiratory valve was then closed and the inspiratory valve opened. The flow of gas through the inspiratory valve was matched to the patient's inspiratory flow rate by adjusting the orifice of the inspiratory valve. This allowed the patient to breathe spontaneously through the ventilator. When a mandatory breath was due the ventilator would wait until the patient began to inspire and then deliver the mandatory breath, synchronising the mandatory breath with the patient's own inspiratory effort or ensuring it occurred when the patient's lungs

were empty. If the patient fails to trigger the ventilator within a preset time interval most machines default to intermittent positive pressure ventilation.

All ventilators with SIMV systems use some form of synchronisation between patient and machine, the exact details varying between machines. All SIMV machines are not equally effective, however, for the time taken for the inspiratory valve to open after the pressure sensor has been triggered varies between machines. During the period between the patient beginning to inspire and the inspiratory valve opening, the patient inspires against a closed valve, so increasing the work of breathing.[20] Machines which have a short lag between the beginning of an inspiratory effort and the inspiratory valve opening are preferred. Although subjectively patients usually appear more comfortable on SIMV than IPPV or IMV, there is no evidence that it reduces morbidity or mortality in intensive care units.[21]

Mandatory minute ventilation

The SIMV systems described above add a preset number of breaths of a preset pattern and volume to the patient's own respiratory efforts. If the patient's spontaneous breaths are providing most of the required minute ventilation, the mandatory breaths may be too large or too frequent. Similarly, if the patient's own respiratory efforts diminish, the mandatory breaths may not be sufficient to provide an adequate minute ventilation. Ideally the ventilator should monitor exhaled volumes and "top up" the patient's respiratory efforts if needed. This is the basis of mandatory minute ventilation. In this mode of ventilation a preset minute volume is selected. If the patient's own respiratory efforts produce a minute ventilation in excess of the preset value, the ventilator does not activate. If the preset minute volume is not achieved the ventilator gives some assistance to the patient, to bring the minute ventilation back to the target value.

The method used to provide ventilatory assistance depends on the design of the ventilator. The Ohmeda CPU1 and Engström Erica will provide synchronised mandatory breaths of a preset tidal volume at an increasing frequency as the patient's own respiratory efforts diminish. The Hamilton Veolar uses a different approach and provides increasing inspiratory pressure support (see below) as the patient's own efforts decrease. Whichever method is used, the machines ensure that the patient always receives a predetermined

11

minute volume. While theoretically attractive the technique has not been widely adopted. The system works well if the patient's respiratory rate is relatively normal, but if the patient develops rapid, shallow breathing the ventilator will measure an adequate minute ventilation even though the bulk of the ventilation will be delivered to anatomical deadspace and so will not contribute to carbon dioxide elimination.

Assist-control

This mode of ventilation was once popular in the United States but was little used in Europe. It is simply intermittent positive pressure ventilation, with each breath triggered by the patient, the pattern of the breath determined by the ventilator.

Inspiratory pressure support

One of the most recent methods of ventilation to be widely used is inspiratory pressure support. It was first introduced in 1981 on Siemens Servo 900C and Engström Erica ventilators. It provides graded assistance with every breath and is similar to the anaesthetist providing ventilatory assistance by squeezing the reservoir bag as the patient inspires. When the patient initiates a breath, the ventilator raises the airway pressure to a preset value. The positive airway pressure provides some of the energy needed to expand the lung, and the efforts of the patient provide the rest. At the end of inspiration the positive airway pressure is removed to allow unimpeded expiration. Patients can determine their own respiratory rate and, by selecting an appropriate level of positive airway pressure, can be given only the respiratory assistance they actually require. This form of ventilation differs from the assist-control mode where, after the patient triggers the ventilator, a preset pattern of pressure or flow is delivered for a fixed period. In inspiratory pressure support a constant pattern of pressure is applied after the patient triggers the ventilator so that the patient can determine the flow pattern and size of breath. Inspiration is usually terminated when the flow has decreased to a predetermined value (usually 25% of the maximum inspiratory flow rate). There are additional safety mechanisms which terminate the flow if the pressure exceeds the preset value or if inspiration is excessively prolonged.

This method of ventilation has theoretical advantages, because intrathoracic pressures and hence haemodynamic upsets are minimised, assistance is provided with every breath, and the patient only receives the support required. Weaning is performed by gradually decreasing the level of pressure support. There are limited data to suggest that inspiratory support is at least as good as SIMV, if not better, for a variety of acute lung conditions.[22] As with SIMV, machines with minimal delays in the triggering mechanism are preferred to minimise the work of breathing. A very recent development is the use of "flowby" or flow triggers. By passing a continuous stream of gas round the breathing circuit, an inspiratory effort can be detected as a change in flow. This method of triggering further reduces the work of breathing.[23]

Pressure controlled ventilation

In the early days of mechanical ventilation, pressure-limited ventilation was widely used because of fears that pressures above 30 cm H_2O might damage the lungs. This method fell into disfavour, however, because patients with lung disease needed higher inflation pressures and the inflation pressure had to be repeatedly adjusted to maintain a constant minute volume in the presence of changing respiratory compliance and resistance. During the past 10 years, new evidence has accumulated showing that lung damage occurs if pressures greater than 40 cm H_2O are generated during the artificial ventilation of patients with acute lung injury and that this is accentuated if large tidal volumes are also used.[24] In addition, the dangers of hypercarbia have probably been overstated in the past, and modest hypercarbia is probably less dangerous than high inflation pressures.[25] This has resulted in the increased use of pressure controlled ventilation together with permissive hypercarbia in adults. Usually the ventilator is used in a time cycled mode and patients do not interact with the ventilator. An added refinement has been the use of inverse ratio ventilation, where the inspiratory time can be up to four times as long as the expiratory time. The short expiratory time increases mean lung volume by maintaining lung inflation for a greater proportion of the respiratory cycle and by creating an alveolar PEEP by air trapping. The haemodynamic effects are similar to extrinsically applied PEEP. The technique requires careful control because small changes in airway resistance and compliance can produce major alterations in lung volume by altering the time constants that determine the rate at which the lungs empty. The combination of pressure-controlled and inverse ratio ventilation has been advocated for lung diseases where a decreased compliance occurs, such as the adult respiratory distress syndrome.[26] It is not suitable for asthma or conditions leading to a high airway resistance where gas trapping is already present.

Airway pressure release ventilation (APRV) and biphasic positive pressure ventilation (BiPAP)

In both these modes of ventilation the patient breathes spontaneously from a continuous positive airway pressure (CPAP) system. A standing pressure (usually 5–10 cm H_2O) is applied to the patient's airway, either via an endotracheal tube or by using a facemask. This causes the patient to breathe at an elevated mean lung volume which increases arterial PO_2 by maintaining expansion in areas of lung that would otherwise collapse. Providing that the pressure within the system is maintained within ± 2 cm H_2O of the set pressure there is little increase in the work of breathing and indeed work may decrease owing to improved lung mechanics. Carbon dioxide retention may occur when CPAP is used. Carbon dioxide elimination can be augmented by periodically emptying the lungs by deflation to atmospheric pressure (APRV) or to a lower positive pressure (BiPAP). This is achieved by opening a second valve on the expiratory side of the system for 2–4 seconds at a frequency of 2–10 times a minute. With BiPAP the system pressure is reduced to a lower PEEP level rather than atmospheric pressure, the aim being to minimise alveolar collapse during expiration. This facility is now provided as an integral part of the Draeger Evita ventilator. These modes of ventilation are both essentially time-cycled, pressure-controlled ventilation with low pressures and respiratory rates superimposed on spontaneous respiration.

Other methods of assisting gas exchange

There are several modes of ventilation which are still being evaluated. High frequency jet ventilation involves directing brief, frequently repeated pulses of gas (up to 300 per minute) from a high pressure nozzle down the airway. The tidal volumes delivered are small, airway pressures are low and the patient can breathe spontaneously while being ventilated.[27] Interest in this mode of ventilation is waning as it offers no clear clinical advantages, yet carries a small risk of complications related to overinflation of the lung and the use of high pressure gas in the airways.

14

High frequency oscillation techniques oscillate gas in the airways using a piston pump or diaphragm pump. The tidal volumes used are very small, and may be much less than the anatomical deadspace, so gas movement occurs by mechanisms other than tidal exchange. Because of the large size of oscillators needed for adults, this technique has previously been confined to use in infants, but an external oscillator using a cuirass has recently been introduced for adults and children.

There are also two extracorporeal systems in clinical use. In adults with acute respiratory failure extracorporeal membrane oxygenation (ECMO) was largely abandoned after the results of a large trial showed that it did not reduce mortality.[28] In infants with neonatal respiratory distress, however, ECMO seems to be very effective. A remarkable reduction in mortality from this condition following the use of ECMO has been reported in America.[29] In adults, a new approach has been pioneered by Gattinoni in Italy. He started with the hypothesis that artificial ventilation itself can exacerbate acute respiratory failure. Tidal ventilation is required only to remove carbon dioxide, and oxygenation can be maintained in apnoeic patients if the carbon dioxide is removed by an extracorporeal circuit. By removing carbon dioxide with an extracorporeal artificial lung and reducing ventilation to the minimum, he claims to have reduced the mortality from acute respiratory failure.[30]

The extracorporeal systems all require a membrane lung outside the body, with vascular access. Initially bleeding was a serious problem but this has been reduced using heparin-coated tubing and percutaneous cannulation. There are still no published controlled trials comparing this technique with standard methods of treatment. Recently, a gas exchange device has become available which is placed percutaneously into the inferior vena cava. In effect it is an internal membrane lung. This device, called an IVOX (IntraVenous OXygenator), has only limited use as it can only achieve 10–28% of the oxygen and carbon dioxide exchange requirements of the patient.[31]

Conclusion

The distinction between a ventilated patient and a spontaneously breathing patient is becoming increasingly blurred as more sophisticated means of respiratory support are devised. In many cases "respiratory assistance" may be a more appropriate term than

15

"artificial ventilation". The efficacy of many of these ventilatory strategies has not been properly assessed, in terms of patient acceptability or changes in morbidity and mortality. It is still true that the type of ventilator used, provided that its design is satisfactory, is of less importance than the experience of the person using it.

1 Baker AB. Early attempts at expired air respiration, intubation and manual ventilation. In: Atkinson RS, Boulton TB, eds. *The history of anaesthesia.* London: Royal Society of Medicine, 1987:372–4.
2 Kite C. *An essay on the recovery of the apparently dead.* London: Dilly, 1788.
3 Gocrig M, Filos K, Ayisi KW. George Edward Fell and the development of respiratory machines. In: Atkinson, RS, Boulton TB, eds. *The history of anaesthesia.* London: Royal Society of Medicine, 1987:386–93.
4 Rendell-Baker L, Pettis JL. The development of positive pressure ventilators. In: Atkinson RS, Boulton TB, eds. *The history of anaesthesia.* London: The Royal Society of Medicine, 1987:402–21.
5 Crafoord C. Pulmonary ventilation and anesthesia in major chest surgery. *J Thoracic Surg* 1940;**9**:237–53.
6 Samuals MP, Southall DP. Negative extrathoracic pressure in the treatment of respiratory failure in infants and young children. *Br Med J* 1989;**299**:1253–7.
7 Smallwood RW. Ventilators–Reported classifications and their usefulness. *Anaesth Intens Care* 1986;**14**:251–7.
8 Mapleson WW. The effect of lung characteristics on the functioning of artificial ventilators. *Anaesthesia* 1962;**17**:300–14.
9 Mushin WW, Rendell-Baker L, Thompson PW, Mapleson WW. Automatic ventilation of the lungs. Oxford: Blackwells, 1980:312–30.
10 Ingelstedt S, Jonson B, Nordstrom L, Olsson S-G. A servo-controlled ventilator measuring expired minute volume, airway flow and pressure. *Acta Anaesthesiol Scand* 1972;Suppl **47**:9–28.
11 Drinker P, McKhann CF. The use of a new apparatus for prolonged administration of artificial respiration. *JAMA* 1929;**92**:1658–61.
12 Miller-Jones CMH, Williams JH. Sedation for ventilation. A retrospective study of fifty patients. *Anaesthesia* 1980;**35**:1104–7.
13 Merriman HM. The techniques used to sedate ventilated patients. *Intens Care Med* 1981; 7:217–24.
14 Willatts SM. Paralysis for ventilated patients? Yes or No? *Intens Care Med* 1985;**11**:2–4.
15 Watt I, Ledingham IMcA. Mortality amongst multiple trauma patients admitted to an intensive therapy unit. *Anaesthesia* 1984;**39**:973–81.
16 Bion JF, Ledingham IMcA. Sedation in intensive care—a postal survey. *Intens Care Med* 1987;**13**:215–16.
17 Venus B, Smith RA, Mathru M. National survey of methods and criteria used for weaning from mechanical ventilation. *Crit Care Med* 1987;**15**:530–3.
18 Sykes MK, McNicol MW, Campbell EJM. Respiratory failure. Oxford: Blackwells, 1976: 320–2.
19 Carroll GC, Tuman KJ, Braverman B, et al. Minimal positive end-expiratory pressure (PEEP) may be best PEEP. *Chest* 1988;**93**:1020–5.
20 Lemaire F. Weaning from mechanical ventilation. In: Ledingham IMcA, ed. *Recent advances in critical care medicine 3* Edinburgh: Churchill Livingstone, 1988:15–30.
21 Weisman IM, Rinaldo JE, Rogers RM, Sanders MH. State of the art: Intermittent mandatory ventilation. *Am Rev Respir Dis* 1983;**127**:641–7.
22 Kacmarek RM. Inspiratory pressure support: does it make a clinical difference? *Intens Care Med* 1989;**15**:337–9.
23 Cox D, Niblett DJ. Studies on continuous positive airway pressure breathing systems. *Br J Anaesth* 1984;**56**:905–11.
24 Parker JC, Hernandez LA, Peevy KJ. Mechanisms of ventilator induced lung injury. *Crit Care Med* 1993;**21**:131–43.

25 Hickling KG, Henderson SJ, Jackson R. Low mortality associated with low volume pressure limited ventilation with permissive hypercapnia in severe adult respiratory distress syndrome. *Intens Care Med* 1990;**16**:372–7.
26 Marcy TW, Marini JJ. Inverse ratio ventilation in ARDS. Rationale and implementation. *Chest* 1991;**100**:494–504.
27 Smith BE, Hanning CD. Advances in respiratory support. *Br J Anaesth* 1986;**58**:138–50.
28 Zapol WM, Snider MT, Hill JD, *et al.* Extracorporeal membrane oxygenation in severe acute respiratory failure. *JAMA* 1979;**242**:2193–6.
29 Toomasian JM, Snedcor SM, Cornell RG, Cilley RE, Bartlett RH. National experience with extracorporeal membrane oxygenation for newborn respiratory failure. *Trans Am Soc Artif Int Organs* 1988;**34**:140–7.
30 Gattinoni L, Pesenti A, Mascheroni D, *et al.* Low-frequency positive-pressure ventilation with extra-corporeal CO_2 removal in acute respiratory failure. *JAMA* 1986;**256**:881–6.
31 High KM, Snider MT, Richard R, *et al.* Clinical trials of an intravenous oxygenator in patients with Adult Respiratory Distress Syndrome. *Anesthesiology* 1992;**77**:856–63.

2 Indications for mechanical ventilation

JOSÉ PONTE

Mechanical ventilation comprises all types of artificial ventilation in which a mechanical device is used to replace or aid the work normally carried out by the ventilatory muscles. It has been used to treat ventilatory failure since the portable "iron lung" was introduced by Drinker and Shaw in 1929,[1] but only during the Copenhagen polio epidemic in 1952 were the skills of anaesthetists and physicians brought together in a breakthrough which established the lifesaving value and simplicity of intermittent positive pressure ventilation.[2 3] This was an important landmark in the treatment of acute respiratory failure and soon afterwards the benefits of mechanical ventilation in the postoperative period were also demonstrated.[4] Unless otherwise stated, this chapter refers to mechanical ventilation as any form of intermittent positive pressure ventilation, applied through an endotracheal tube, with or without positive end expiratory pressure or allowance for spontaneous breaths.

Mechanical ventilation is indicated where established or impending respiratory failure exists, defined as the inability of the breathing apparatus to maintain normal gas exchange. Respiratory failure may be predominantly due to failure of oxygenation (type I) or to an inability to eliminate carbon dioxide (type II or "ventilatory" failure). Type I failure is usually associated with lung parenchymal disease, alveolar collapse or an increase in lung water. Type II failure can be associated with a lack of ventilatory drive, musculoskeletal disease or neuromuscular blockade but it also occurs in primary pulmonary disorders in which the ventilatory load is excessive relative to capacity (for example severe chronic obstructive airways disease). In principle, mechanical ventilation is indicated predominantly for ventilatory failure (type II).

The majority of patients receiving mechanical ventilation do not have pulmonary disease. They are undergoing surgery under general

18

TABLE 2.1—Main indications for mechanical ventilation in adults

---

Routine anaesthesia and postoperative management of major surgery

Respiratory impairment (parenchymal, airway or chest wall)
Pneumonia, adult respiratory distress syndrome
Asthma, acute exacerbation in chronic bronchitis or emphysema
Lung contusion, chest trauma with flail segment, ruptured diaphragm
Chest wall burns, kyphoscoliosis, cystic fibrosis

Central nervous system or neuromuscular impairment
Drug overdose: narcotics, anaesthetics, barbiturates
Intracranial bleed, trauma, meningoencephalitis, tumours, infarction
Brain oedema, raised intracranial pressure
Central hypoventilation, status epilepticus, tetanus, rabies
Polyneuritis, Guillain–Barré, Lambert–Eaton
Myasthenia gravis, paralysing poisons, myopathies

Circulatory failure
Cardiac arrest, severe shock (sepsis or other causes)
Left ventricular failure (pulmonary oedema)

---

anaesthesia with the aid of neuromuscular blocking drugs. Outside the operating theatre, most patients receive mechanical ventilation in the intensive therapy unit. Surveys carried out in nonspecialised intensive therapy units in several industrialised countries have shown that most patients requiring mechanical ventilation are in the postoperative stage (about 65% of all patients) following cardiac, aortic, neuro or other major surgery; they rarely need mechanical ventilation for more than 24 hours. The other major groups requiring ventilation are patients with head or chest trauma (about 10%), poisoning (about 8%) and those who are critically ill with severe primary respiratory disease (about 13%).[5–8] A few patients receive mechanical ventilation at home or in specialised institutions; they are considered separately in chapter 5.

Indications for mechanical ventilation in adults are listed in table 2.1. Indications for mechanical ventilation in anaesthesia, in the postoperative period, in neonates and in organ donation are outside the scope of this chapter. Mechanical ventilation should be used only when it is strictly necessary since there are many inherent risks.[9] Indeed, ventilation may unnecessarily prolong the distress of terminal disease and the benefits of its use should, therefore, be carefully weighed against the disadvantages. The basic "recipe" for setting up mechanical ventilation in a patient without lung

19

TABLE 2.2—Basic "recipe" for setting up mechanical ventilation in an adult without pulmonary pathology and with a normal metabolic rate

Airway
Access via oral or nasal cuffed endotracheal tube or cuffed tracheostomy tube

Ventilator
Set tidal volume (VT) at 8 ml/kg body weight
Set rate (RR) at 12–14 breaths/min; minute volume ($= VT \times RR$) should be 80–90 ml/kg body weight
Set ratio of inspiratory:expiratory time to 1:3; peak inflation pressure should not exceed 30 cm H_2O
Provide humidification of inspired gas mixture
Set O_2 concentration at 30–60%
Set alarms for:
• ventilator disconnection
• peak inspiratory pressure >30 cm H_2O
• oxygen inspired concentration 25–60%

Patient
Ensure analgesia and sedation: mandatory if patient is paralysed (neuromuscular blockers only when strictly necessary, for example, head injuries or tetanus) use propofol, opiates or benzodiazepines
Monitor effects of intermittent positive pressure ventilation on circulation and gastric distension
Check blood gases regularly (2–4 hourly) and after changing any of the ventilator settings:
• adjust minute volume according to arterial carbon dioxide tension
• adjust inspired oxygen concentration and positive end expiratory pressure according to arterial oxygen tension
Institute basic nursing care for the unconscious patient:
• regular routine observations, turning on bed, mouth wash
• regular check for bilateral breath sounds and expansion of both lungs, there is a risk of endobronchial intubation, pneumothorax or accumulation of secretions
• regular check for state of consciousness, need of pain relief, and sedation
Chest radiograph on alternate days to check for:
• positions of endotracheal tube, intravascular canuli, nasogastric tube
• pleural or pulmonary abnormalities

pathology is given in table 2.2. Guidelines for standards of care of ventilated patients are available.[10]

Benefits of mechanical ventilation

The principal benefit of mechanical ventilation is the control gained over the airway and over the work of breathing. The ventilator replaces the work of exhausted or temporarily inadequate respiratory muscles. The ability to remove secretions from upper airways (by simple suction or aided by fibreoptic bronchoscopy) may be advantageous and additional measures, such as positive end expiratory pressure or effective aerosol delivery, may be instituted in certain patients. Ventilation also allows large doses of narcotic analgesics or neuromuscular blocking agents to be used where clinically indicated (in tetanus, for example, or in any situation where reflex coughing and contraction of the expiratory muscles impairs effective ventilation). Clinical situations in which mechanical ventilation may be of benefit are listed in table 2.1.

Risks and side effects of mechanical ventilation

Some dangers of mechanical ventilation apply to all patients. It is not possible to establish effective, long term ventilation without securing a sealed connection with the airway via an endotracheal or tracheostomy tube; the insertion of this tube, however, requires either general or local anaesthesia with its attendant risks.

Anaesthesia

The risks associated with the anaesthesia needed for endotracheal intubation include: myocardial depression caused by general or local anaesthetic drugs; aspiration of gastric contents; a further fall in arterial oxygen tension, especially if intubation is difficult; an idiosyncratic reaction to the anaesthetic drugs; and reflex worsening of bronchoconstriction following tracheal intubation or suction of secretions. These risks are not substantially reduced if a topical local anaesthetic is used instead of general anaesthetic for the intubation of the trachea.

Sedation and paralysis

Intermittent positive pressure ventilation through a nasal or an orotracheal tube is poorly tolerated without some sedation. Sometimes paralysing drugs are also required, especially in neurological disease (for example, status epilepticus) or trauma. The choice of methods and indications for sedation are dealt with in more detail in chapter 3. In general, the ideal sedative should be very short acting, it should be given by constant intravenous infusion and should have minimal side effects, especially on the circulation. The available sedatives all have important side effects. The opiates are complicated by tolerance and paralysis of the gut (with consequent delay in absorption) and their prolonged respiratory depressant effects delay weaning from the ventilator. Barbiturates and chlor-

21

methiazole present similar problems and also cause myocardial depression. Increasing doses of benzodiazepines are often required because of tolerance, leading to a build up of active metabolites and prolonged depressant effects on the central nervous system, which last for days after stopping administration. Of the established anaesthetics, only two relatively recently introduced drugs, currently under assessment for long term sedation, have potential as sedatives in the intensive therapy unit: propofol,[11] an intravenous anaesthetic and isoflurane,[12] a volatile inhalation anaesthetic. They are both short acting agents, with minimal cumulative effects and their cardiovascular and respiratory effects at sedative doses are mild in the fit patient; however, the cardiac depressant effects of these two drugs may be important in the patient with poor myocardial function. There is a wide choice of suitable neuromuscular blocking drugs: vecuronium and atracurium have minimal side effects and are sufficiently short acting to allow rapid regulation of the state of paralysis. All staff in the intensive therapy unit should be aware that neuromuscular blocking agents have no sedative effects and that patients may be awake and paralysed if sedation is not prescribed. Another danger of paralysis is the inability of the patient to make spontaneous breathing efforts should there be an accidental ventilator disconnection.

Equipment failure

The risks of equipment failure include accidental disconnection of the ventilator, undetected leaks or malfunction of the endotracheal tube, all leading to alveolar hypoventilation. Barotrauma to the lungs may occur if high inflation pressures are applied to the airway, leading to pneumothorax, pneumomediastinum, pneumopericardium, and subcutaneous emphysema. Tracheal burns may occur if heated humidifiers are used. Oxygen toxicity may occur if the inspired oxygen is higher than 60% for a prolonged period of time.

Hyperinflation

Hyperinflation not associated with equipment failure occurs in patients with severe acute bronchospasm or chronic airflow limitation with increased functional residual capacity. Intermittent positive pressure ventilation may lead to very high intrathoracic pressures with adverse effects on cardiac output and increased risk of barotrauma.

Cardiovascular effects

Intermittent positive pressure ventilation causes an increase in mean intrathoracic pressure, especially if positive end expiratory pressure is used, leading to a fall in cardiac output due to direct mechanical interference with the heart and large veins. These effects are unimportant in the relatively fit patient undergoing elective surgery, but may not be tolerated in the severely ill patient with hypovolaemia or with increased airway resistance.[13-15] There are also indirect cardiovascular effects of intermittent positive pressure ventilation mediated through reflexes of the autonomic nervous system and through hormone release or changes in blood gases. The predominant direct adverse effects of intermittent positive pressure ventilation on the right heart are a reduction in venous return (preload) and an increase in pulmonary vascular resistance (afterload). Right ventricular performance may also be adversely affected if the right ventricular ejection fraction is less than 0·4.[16] The direct effects on the left heart are less marked and less well established, the widely held view being that both pulmonary venous return (preload) and afterload decrease. This effect on left ventricular afterload is due to a fall in ventricular transmural pressure because of the increase in intrathoracic pressure (this also applies to the right ventricle).[17] This mechanism provides a form of "assistance" to ventricular work which may be beneficial in cardiac failure.[15 18] The reflex responses are complex, depending on multiple neural and chemical feedback loops.[19] The neural reflexes are mediated initially by the vagus nerve affecting predominantly the heart rate, but stronger reflexes involve the whole sympathetic system[20] affecting vascular resistances and circulating catecholamines. The reflexes originate from lung and atrial stretch receptors and from the arterial baroreceptors and chemoreceptors (the latter only if arterial carbon dioxide tension falls or arterial oxygen tension rises in response to intermittent positive pressure ventilation). The humoral reflex response to intermittent positive pressure ventilation includes an increase in antidiuretic hormone and renin-angiotensin and a decrease in atrial natriuretic peptide, which may be partly responsible for the sodium retention seen in ventilated patients[21]; the changes in catecholamines are partly mediated by changes in arterial carbon dioxide tension. The pattern of circulatory changes is variable; the predominant effect is a decrease in both cardiac output (typically by 25%) and arterial

23

blood pressure, an increase in heart rate and a slight increase in systemic vascular resistance; right and left atrial pressures increase relative to atmospheric pressure (transmural pressures *decrease*). There is evidence of decreased splanchnic blood flow and increased splanchnic congestion during mechanical ventilation with positive end expiratory pressure.[22] This pattern is often modified by blood gas changes associated with mechanical ventilation because of the powerful stimulant effects of carbon dioxide on the sympathetic system.

Finally, the venous drainage from the head is slightly impaired by the increased intrathoracic pressure associated with mechanical ventilation. Normally, this effect is not important but it may aggravate an increased intracranial pressure, especially if high inflation pressures are applied.

Criteria for initiation of mechanical ventilation

Despite the risks listed above, mechanical ventilation is a lifesaving procedure in patients developing acute severe respiratory failure secondary to reversible conditions, examples are severe pneumonia, severe bronchospasm, neuromuscular syndromes involving respiratory muscles, head or chest trauma, pulmonary oedema secondary to heart failure, poisoning, and septic shock. In most cases, the indications for mechanical ventilation are clear cut and ventilation is seldom needed for more than 48 hours.

In general, mechanical ventilation is rarely indicated unless there is respiratory failure, exceptions are the postoperative period following major surgery and the management of raised intracranial pressure. There are circumstances, however, where the indications for mechanical ventilation are less clear.[23 24] In some centres, for example, mechanical ventilation is routinely instituted before the onset of type II respiratory failure in the adult respiratory distress syndrome, although there is no evidence that this alters the course or the final outcome of the syndrome.[25]

Even when acute respiratory failure is clearly life threatening, mechanical ventilation may not be indicated if the underlying condition is terminal malignancy, advanced AIDS or severe chronic airflow limitation. It is often difficult to predict whether it will be possible to wean these patients from the ventilator and published figures from various centres indicate that the mortality, even when ventilated, is very high.[7 26] Because of the poor outcome and the high human and material costs of managing mechanical ventilation in this group of patients,[27] it may be appropriate to withhold mechanical ventilation. This decision should always be made by a senior physician, taking into account the present wishes of the fully conscious patient or the known wishes of the unconscious patient. When dealing with an unconscious patient the views of the closest relatives and of the medical and nursing staff directly involved in the management should also be considered. Where there is doubt, it is ethically more acceptable to withdraw treatment later rather than withhold it at the moment of crisis.[26 27] All possible measures should be used in these patients to postpone the need for ventilation, for example, the use of doxapram if there is inadequate respiratory drive, continuous positive airway pressure if the main problem is airway collapse and nasal intermittent positive pressure ventilation, which may be well tolerated over short periods, obviating the need for endotracheal intubation.[28]

It is often difficult to define the precise moment when ventilation should be started. Despite 70 years of worldwide experience with mechanical ventilation, there are no exact criteria on which to base a decision.[23] In the past 25 years, however, guidelines have evolved from a consensus of opinion among physicians and anaesthetists. A set of physiological variables with a range of critical values which have been proposed by several authors are given in table 2.3. Since these critical values are empirical, merely representing the accumulated experience of clinicians,[7 23 26] the decision to ventilate must rest firmly on the clinical assessment of the patient. For example, the presence of rapidly worsening respiratory variables is more important than a single critical value being exceeded; fatigue and exhaustion cannot be easily quantified and the judgement of an experienced clinician, who takes into account the quality of the monitoring and the nursing supervision, is essential. It is generally accepted, however, that the attainment of any of the critical values in table 2.3 is associated with terminal respiratory failure unless mechanical ventilation is instituted.[13] The algorithm shown in figure 2.1 provides a simple guide to the sequence of decisions leading up to starting mechanical ventilation in respiratory failure. The diagnosis of life threatening respiratory failure (box 1) may be made on clinical grounds alone: for example, if the patient is unconscious and cyanosed or has suffered respiratory arrest the decision to ventilate may be reached within a matter of seconds, following the direct path from assess to IPPV.

TABLE 2.3—Critical values* of physiological variables widely accepted as part of the criteria for administering mechanical ventilation to adult patients (normal ranges in parentheses)

Ventilatory mechanics

Respiratory rate (breaths/min)	>35	(12–20)
Tidal volume (VT; ml/kg)	<3	(5–7)
Minute ventilation (l/min)	<3 or >20	(6–10)
Vital capacity (VC; ml/kg)	<10–15†	(65–75)
Peak expiratory flow (PEF)	<50% of normal	
FEV$_1$ (ml/kg)	<10	(50–70)
Maximum negative inspiratory pressure (cm H$_2$O)	>20–25†	(75–100)
VD:VT ratio	>0·6	(0·25–0·4)

Blood gases

Pao$_2$ (kPa with 60% inspired oxygen)	<8	
P(A−a)O$_2$ (kPa with 100% inspired oxygen)	>46–60†‡	(3·3–8·6)
Paco$_2$ (kPa)	>6·7–8†§	(4·6–6·0)

Circulatory variables

Cardiac output (l/min)	<2	
Cardiac index (l/min/m^2)	<1·2	(2–3·5)

* The values in this table summarise those appearing in the current literature.[5-7 20 21 23] Consequently, they are only approximate and VT, VC and FEV$_1$ are not given in relation to age and gender.
† Range of published values.[7 20 23]
‡ After at least 10 minutes of continuous 100% inspired oxygen.
§ In patients without metabolic acidosis or chronic hypercapnia.
VD, dead space; PaO$_2$, arterial oxygen tension; P(A−a)O$_2$, alveolar–arterial oxygen tension difference.

Ideally, severe respiratory failure should be anticipated and the decision to ventilate should be made before more than one of the critical values in table 2.3 is exceeded. Severe dyspnoea, restlessness and exhaustion are in themselves good indicators for initiating ventilation when the underlying clinical condition is not expected to improve within 1–2 hours. Patients with impending acute respiratory failure need frequent and expert monitoring in an intensive care setting so that a decision to ventilate can be made at the appropriate time. Admission to the intensive therapy unit should therefore be arranged before mechanical ventilation is needed, since a delay in the decision to ventilate may trigger a sequence of irreversible events, including multiple organ failure and cerebral oedema. Furthermore, the risks associated with sedation and endotracheal intubation increase as the clinical state of the patient deteriorates. The patient is too often allowed to deteriorate too far in the general medical or surgical ward before being admitted to

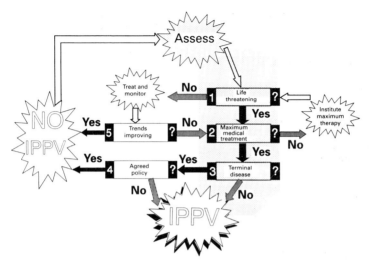

FIG 2.1—A simple guide to help decide when to institute mechanical ventilation in life threatening respiratory failure. The five boxes represent decisions based on clinical assessment, each has two outlets; yes or no.

the intensive care unit. On the other hand, the usual consensus among physicians and surgeons, because of the high costs and the fierce competition for beds, is that admission to the intensive care unit is not warranted until mechanical ventilation is essential. This deadlock, with obvious disadvantages for the patient, can be resolved only if clear policies for admission to the intensive care unit are agreed among the senior clinicians concerned. Scoring systems that help to predict the probability of survival of severely ill patients[7 8] may be helpful in defining such an admission policy.

Difficult patients

Some clinical situations deserve separate discussion because of their special risks and difficulties.

Failure to oxygenate

Hypoxaemia without hypercarbia (type I respiratory failure) may persist and deteriorate despite medical treatment, including continuous positive airway pressure and 100% inspired oxygen. The usual cause is a massive shunt, secondary to bilateral consolidation, adult respiratory distress syndrome or pulmonary oedema. In the

27

awake patient, severe hypoxaemia greatly increases ventilatory drive leading to hyperventilation and eventual respiratory muscle fatigue and exhaustion. Hypoxaemia causes multiple organ dysfunction, including skeletal muscle dysfunction. In addition to treating the cause of hypoxaemia the aim of management should be to minimise the total oxygen demand of the body and to maximise the transfer of oxygen from the inspired gas to the tissues. The total oxygen demand can be reduced by abolishing muscle activity through muscle paralysis and by reducing body temperature. Mechanical ventilation may be life saving in these circumstances because it reduces or abolishes the work of breathing and allows the use of neuromuscular blockers to prevent shivering and other skeletal muscle activity. In addition to taking over from exhausted respiratory muscles, mechanical ventilation also allows better expansion of the lungs, more effective application of continuous pressure and more effective suction of secretions from the airway, including the performance of therapeutic bronchoscopy. In the case of cardiogenic pulmonary oedema, effective continuous positive pressure also helps to reverse the pressure gradient across the alveolar membrane consequently reducing extravascular lung water. The complications of mechanical ventilation, outlined earlier in this chapter, should not be underestimated. The risks involved with anaesthesia and intubation of the trachea are especially high in severe hypoxaemia because it is almost certain that ventilation will need to be interrupted for a short period of time, temporarily worsening oxygenation.

Acute severe asthma

Respiratory failure is accompanied by chest hyperinflation, impaired diaphragm function, tachypnoea and marked use of accessory muscles. When intermittent positive pressure ventilation is applied, inflation pressure can be very high (>50 cm H_2O) with a very steep upward slope with each inflation, indicating very low chest compliance. The overinflated lung operates in a region of the pressure–volume curve where great changes of pressure are needed to produce small volume changes. These high intrathoracic pressures may have a marked effect on the circulation, causing a fall in cardiac output; the risk of barotrauma is high. When intermittent positive pressure ventilation is indicated in the exhausted, rapidly deteriorating patient it should not initially aim at correcting $Paco_2$; values up to 9 kPa are acceptable. Maximum medical treatment should be maintained for as long as the severe bronchospasm lasts, following established guidelines.[29] Tidal volume should be small (<10 ml/kg) and the ratio of inspiratory to expiratory time must be low (<1:3), allowing maximum time for the lungs to deflate in expiration.[30] Maximum inspired oxygen concentration (100%) should be used to maintain oxygenation during the short period of life threatening respiratory failure. Saturated humidification of inspired gases, warmed to body temperature, is essential. The use of positive end expiratory pressure is generally contraindicated. A more detailed review of this subject can be found elsewhere.[31]

Patients at special risk from barotrauma

A proportion of patients with chronic respiratory failure have bullous emphysema and intermittent positive pressure ventilation in these patients considerably increases the risk of barotrauma. Positive end expiratory pressure is usually contraindicated and inflation pressures should not exceed 40 cm H_2O with a maximum inspiratory to expiratory ratio of 1:2, even if the patient remains underventilated (maintaining oxygenation by raising F_IO_2). The patient should be closely monitored for signs of tension pneumothorax (sudden increase in inflation pressure, tachycardia, and fall in blood pressure) and equipment should be ready for the insertion of a chest drain. When bullae burst and drains are inserted, the difficult problems of bronchopleural fistulae may supervene.

Patients with stiff lungs

Stiff lungs are usually the result of chronic interstitial disease or the adult respiratory distress syndrome, secondary to cardiovascular shock, acid aspiration or trauma. Maximal medical treatment may include the use of inhaled nitric oxide and the instillation of exogenous surfactant into the bronchial tree.[32] Mechanical ventilation is used to replace the excessive work demanded of the respiratory muscles during the acute phase; high inflation pressures are needed, with positive end expiratory pressure if necessary to maintain oxygenation, provided cardiac output is not severely compromised. In terms of peripheral oxygen delivery, a normal cardiac output with a PaO_2 of 6 kPa is better than half the normal cardiac output with a PaO_2 of 12 kPa. Low PaO_2 values are acceptable if the haemoglobin content of blood is near normal and cardiac output can reflexly rise above normal (haemodynamic monitoring and oxygen delivery are discussed in chapter 3). The high inflation pressures sometimes necessary in these patients lead to other difficulties, including barotrauma and maintaining an adequate seal of the endotracheal tube without overinflating the cuff and damaging the trachea. It is impossible to predict accurately whether the respiratory muscles will be able to cope with chronically stiff lungs after the acute phase has passed.

Special mechanical ventilation techniques

The "nuts and bolts" of ventilators and modalities of mechanical ventilation are reviewed in chapter 1. Intermittent positive pressure ventilation, with or without positive end expiratory pressure, is the modality of mechanical ventilation best suited to anaesthesia, postoperative ventilation, cardiopulmonary resuscitation, and the majority of non-surgical admissions to the intensive care unit. Modifications of the original technique, which allow spontaneous or assisted breaths, are often used in intensive care units. The problems of weaning are dealt with in chapter 4. Two special techniques merit further discussion because of their potential application in difficult cases.

High frequency ventilation

High frequency ventilation is defined in chapter 1. It provides small inflations, usually at a rate of 200–300 breaths per minute, by means of a special ventilator. The technique can maintain adequate gas exchange with lower peak inflation pressures than occur with conventional ventilation, but it produces similar or higher mean airway pressures, offering clear advantages in only a very few situations.[33] There are unresolved problems with the equipment, such as the monitoring of airway pressures, and the reliable humidification of gases. It has been suggested that high frequency ventilation has advantages over conventional mechanical ventilation in the treatment of persistent bronchopleural fistula[34] and respiratory failure associated with cardiac failure[35]; both these claims have been disputed.[36 37]

Differential ventilation

Differential ventilation allows ventilation of each lung with different gas mixtures or different pressure–time settings. It requires either a double lumen endotracheal tube or two cuffed bronchial tubes. Two synchronised ventilators are also needed. Experience with this technique is limited; the published evidence is based on case reports in patients with unilateral lung pathology and work on experimental animals. Reported uses of differential ventilation include the treatment of patients with persistent bronchopleural fistula or unilateral bullae and cases where copious secretions from one lung are affecting the function of the normal lung. If high fractional inspired oxygen or high inflation pressures are needed, because of unilateral disease, the "good" lung can be spared the risk of oxygen toxicity or excessive inflation pressures by differential ventilation.[38] A recent review of differential ventilation is available.[39]

Special monitoring

It is difficult to adjust ventilator settings and assess the beneficial effects of mechanical ventilation without monitoring gas exchange.

In general, the minute volume is adjusted to maintain the arterial or end tidal carbon dioxide tension at the desired level, usually 5 kPa, or 3–4 kPa in raised intracranial pressure. The inspired oxygen concentration should be the lowest possible above 35% capable of producing an arterial oxygen tension greater than 10 kPa. Preference should be given to the use of positive end expiratory pressure (5–10 cm H_2O) against increasing inspired oxygen concentration to achieve an acceptable arterial oxygen tension, if this is not contraindicated by the risk of bronchopleural leakage or by existing lung hyperinflation.

The aim of gas exchange in the lung is to allow adequate delivery of oxygen and removal of carbon dioxide from the tissues. Thus, in the ventilated patient attention must be paid to the other variables that determine oxygen delivery; the haemoglobin content of the blood and the cardiac output. An adult middle-aged patient with a normal cardiac reserve and a normal haemoglobin level can easily tolerate arterial oxygen tensions of 6·5–7 kPa for days or weeks without developing multiple organ failure. If the cardiac output and/or the oxygen carrying capacity ("usable" haemoglobin) are reduced, oxygen delivery is compromised and hypoxaemia is not well tolerated. As a consequence, anaerobic metabolism occurs in the tissues and lactic acid accumulates. Blood gas analysis shows increasing metabolic acidaemia, quantified by the "base excess" calculation. Values more negative than −8 mmol/l should lead to immediate steps to improve oxygen delivery, such as increasing the arterial oxygen tension (if possible), blood transfusion if the

31

haemoglobin content is lower than 8 g/dl, and infusion of inotropic agents if the cardiac index is less than 1·5.

If the amount of oxygen delivered to the tissues is inadequate more oxygen will be extracted from arterial blood during its passage through the tissues, thereby reducing the oxygen content of venous blood. Consequently, the proportion of oxyhaemoglobin in mixed venous blood falls below its normal value of 70–75%. In addition to monitoring arterial blood gases (including base excess) and cardiac output (by thermodilution or dye-dilution) the continuous monitoring of mixed venous blood haemoglobin saturation may be indicated, using a fibreoptic oximeter incorporated in a flow-directed catheter with the tip placed in the pulmonary artery. Provided there is no important central or peripheral left to right shunt, mixed venous blood saturation monitoring provides an excellent guide for the management of oxygen delivery.[40]

1 Drinker P, Shaw LA. An apparatus for the prolonged administration of artificial respiration. I. A design for adults and children. *J Clin Invest*, 1929;7:229–47.
2 Lassen HCA. The epidemic of poliomyelitis in Copenhagen, 1952. *Proc R Soc Med*, 1954; 47:67–71.
3 Ibsen B. The anaesthetist's viewpoint on the treatment of respiratory complications in poliomyelitis during the epidemic in Copenhagen, 1952. *Proc R Soc Med*, 1954;47:72–4.
4 Björk VO, Engström CG. The treatment of ventilatory insufficiency after pulmonary resection with tracheostomy and prolonged artificial ventilation. *J Thorac Cardiovasc Surg*, 1955;30:356–67.
5 Pontoppidan H, Geffin B, Lowenstein E. Acute respiratory failure in the adult. *N Engl J Med*, 1972;287:690–8, 743–52, 799–806.
6 Petty TL, Lakshminarayan S, Sahn SA, Zwillich CW, Nett LM. Intensive respiratory care unit; review of ten years experience. *JAMA*, 1975;233:34–7.
7 Knaus WA. Prognosis with mechanical ventilation: the influence of disease, severity of disease, age, and chronic health status on survival from an acute illness. *Am Rev Respir Dis*, 1989;140:S8–S13.
8 Rowan KM, Kerr JH, Major E, McPherson K, Short A, Vessey MP. Intensive Care Society's APACHE II study in Britain and Ireland. I: Variations in case mix of adult admissions to general intensive care units and impact on outcome. *BMJ*, 1993;307:972–81.
9 Zwillich CW, Pierson DJ, Creagh CE, Sutton FD, Schatz E, Petty TL. Complications of assisted ventilation: a prospective study of 354 consecutive episodes. *Am J Med*, 1974; 57:161–70.
10 Task Force on Guidelines; Society of Critical Care Medicine. Guidelines for standards of care for patients with acute respiratory failure on mechanical ventilatory support. *Critical Care Med*,1991;19:275–8.
11 Newman LH, McDonald JC, Wallace PGM, Ledingham IM. Propofol for sedation in intensive care. *Anaesthesia*, 1987;42:929–37.
12 Kong KL, Willatts SM, Prys-Roberts C. Isoflurane compared with midazolam for sedation in the intensive care unit. *Br Med J*, 1989;298:1277–80.
13 Cassidy SS, Eschenbacher WL, Robertson CH, Nixon JV, Bloomqvist G, Johnson RL. Cardiovascular effects of positive-pressure ventilation in normal subjects. *J Appl Physiol*, 1979;47:453–61.
14 Luce JM. The cardiovascular effects of mechanical ventilation and positive end expiratory pressure. *JAMA*, 1984;252:807–11.
15 Wallis TW, Robotham JL, Compean R, Kindred MK. Mechanical heart-lung interaction with positive end-expiratory pressure. *J Appl Physiol*, 1983;54:1039–47.

16 Imai T, Uchiyama M, Maruyama N, Yoshikawa D, Fujita T. Influence of constant sustained positive airway pressure on right ventricular performance. *Int Care Med*, 1993;**19**:8–12.
17 Cassidy SS, Mitchell JH. Effects of positive pressure breathing on right and left ventricular preload and afterload. *Fed Proc*,1981;**40**:2178–81.
18 Permutt S. Circulatory effects of weaning from mechanical ventilation: the importance of transdiaphragmatic pressure. *Anesthesiology*, 1988;**69**:157–60.
19 Stinnett HO. Altered cardiovascular reflex responses during positive pressure breathing. *Fed Proc*, 1981;**40**:2182–7.
20 Feuk U, Jakobson S, Norlén K. The effects of alpha adrenergic blockade on central haemodynamics and regional blood flows during positive pressure ventilation: an experimental study in the pig. *Acta Anaesthesiol Scand*, 1987;**31**:748–55.
21 Kharasch ED, Yeo KT, Kenny MA, Buffington CH. Atrial natriuretic factor may mediate the renal effects of PEEP ventilation. *Anesthesiology*, 1988;**69**:862–9.
22 Fujita Y. Effects of PEEP on splanchnic hemodynamics and blood volume. *Acta Anaesthesiol Scand*, 1993;**37**:427–31.
23 Grum CM, Morganroth ML. Initiating mechanical ventilation. *J Int Care Med*, 1988;**3**: 6–20.
24 Snider GL. Historical perspective on mechanical ventilation: from simple life support system to ethical dilemma. *Am Rev Respir Dis*, 1989;**140**:S2–S7.
25 Pepe PE, Hudson LD, Carrico CJ. Early application of positive end-expiratory pressure in patients at risk for the adult respiratory distress syndrome. *N Engl J Med*, 1984;**311**: 281–6.
26 Hudson LD. Survival data in patients with acute and chronic lung disease requiring mechanical ventilation. *Am Rev Respir Dis*, 1989;**140**:S19–S24.
27 Rosen RL, Bone RC. Economics of mechanical ventilation. *Clin Chest Med*, 1988;**9**:163–9.
28 Elliott MW, Steven MH, Phillips GD, Branthwaite MA. Non-invasive mechanical ventilation for acute respiratory failure. *Br Med J*, 1990;**300**:358–60.
29 British Thoracic Society and others. Guidelines for the management of asthma: a summary. *BMJ*, 1993;**306**:776–82.
30 Tuxen DV, Lane S. The effects of ventilatory pattern on hyperinflation, airway pressures, and circulation in mechanical ventilation of patients with severe air-flow obstruction. *Am Rev Respir Dis*, 1987;**136**:872–9.
31 Finfer SR, Garrard CS. Ventilatory support in asthma. *Br J Hosp Med*, 1993;**49**:357–60.
32 Beale R, Grover ER, Smithies M, Bihari D. Acute respiratory distress syndrome ("ARDS"): no more than a severe acute lung injury? *Br Med J*, 1993;**307**:1335–9.
33 MacIntyre N. New forms of mechanical ventilation in the adult. *Clin Chest Med*, 1988;**9**: 47–54.
34 Gallagher TJ, Klain MM, Carlon GC. Present status of high frequency ventilation. *Crit Care Med*, 1982;**10**:613–17.
35 Fuscardi J, Rouby JJ, Barakat T, Mal H, Godet G, Viars P. Hemodynamic effects of high-frequency jet ventilation in patients with and without circulatory shock. *Anesthesiology*, 1986;**65**:485–91.
36 Bishop MJ, Benson MS, Sato P, Pierson DJ. Comparison of high-frequency jet ventilation with conventional mechanical ventilation for bronchopleural fistula. *Anesth Analg*, 1987; **66**:833–8.
37 Crimi G, Conti G, Bufi M, et al. High frequency jet ventilation (HFJV) has no better haemodynamic tolerance than controlled mechanical ventilation (CMV) in cardiogenic shock. *Int Care Med*, 1988;**14**:359–63.
38 Carlon GC, Ray C, Klein R, Goldiner PL, Miodowwnik S. Criteria for selective positive end-expiratory pressure and independent synchronized ventilation of each lung. *Chest*, 1978;**74**:501–7.
39 Adoumie R, Shennib H, Brown R, Slinger P, Chiu RCJ. Differential lung ventilation – applications beyond the operating room. *J Thoracic Cardiovasc Surg*, 1993;**105**:229–33.
40 Beale PL, MacMichan JC, Marsh HM, et al. Continuous monitoring of mixed venous oxygen saturation in critically ill patients. *Anesth Analg*, 1982;**61**:513–8.

3 General care of the ventilated patient in the intensive care unit

M R HAMILTON-FARRELL, GILLIAN C HANSON

Airway and tracheostomy

Patients whose conscious level is impaired often require an artificial aid to maintain a clear airway. An oral (Guedel) airway may temporarily be sufficient, and it allows the passage of a suction catheter alongside. A nasopharyngeal airway is more comfortable, and may permit passage of fine catheters through the larynx; this can be traumatic, however, if repeated too often.

An endotracheal tube or tracheostomy is necessary: to secure the airway against laryngeal obstruction; to provide a route for artificial ventilation; to allow suction of bronchial secretions; and to protect the lungs against aspiration of pharyngeal and gastric contents (table 3.1).

Early problems with endotracheal tubes include misplacement into the oesophagus, or a mainstem bronchus.[1] Subsequent flexion, extension or turning of the neck may displace the tube tip. Other complications are aspiration past an incompletely inflated balloon cuff, oropharyngeal mucous membrane injuries, paralysis and granulomas of vocal cords, and laryngotracheal stenosis.[2] Accidental and self-extubation are risks, especially with young children,[3] and the inflated cuff may damage the larynx as it passes through (table 3.2).

TABLE 3.1—Indications for endotracheal intubation

- To obtain an airway secure from obstruction
- To provide a route for artificial ventilation
- To allow suction of bronchial secretions
- To protect the lungs from aspiration of pharyngeal and gastric contents

34

TABLE 3.2—Complications of endotracheal intubation

Early
- Misplacement into oesophagus or mainstem bronchus
- Aspiration of pharyngeal and gastric contents past a deflated cuff
- Oropharyngeal mucous membrane injuries

Late
- Vocal cord paralysis and granulomata
- Tracheal mucosal trauma from suctioning
- Paranasal sinusitis (nasal tubes only)
- Sepsis (bronchial or intrapulmonary)
- Tracheal stenosis

Although the oral route is often easier for intubation, nasal endotracheal tubes have the advantage of avoiding trauma to the mouth, and of being more comfortable for the awake patient. They are also longer and narrower than oral tubes, and occasionally present problems with suctioning. They may be associated with paranasal sinusitis, a complication made more likely by the simultaneous use of steroids.[4-7]

The use of plastic materials, standardised connector sizes, and uniform fixation techniques have helped to reduce some of the problems of endotracheal tubes.[8] The introduction of high volume, low pressure cuffs may help to prevent tracheal mucosal damage, though other factors are also important. Periods of hypotension and sepsis may compromise the mucosal blood supply, and frequent changes of tube may also damage the larynx. Tracheal mucosal damage is associated with local sepsis.[9]

Ulceration and granulomas of the vocal cords are found in many patients following 5–14 days of intubation.[10] Vocal cord paresis may also be found.[11] These complications are associated with laryngeal oedema, and usually resolve in the days and weeks after extubation. Tracheostomy will prevent these lesions.

Suctioning may cause mucosal damage, and ciliary action may be impaired by the frequent use of high vacuum suction apparatus working through a single end-placed hole.[12 13] Pneumothorax may also be caused by suctioning, especially in young children. Neonates are liable to develop subglottic oedema and stenosis after intubation.[14 15] Subsequent hoarseness and inspiratory stridor may be precipitated by an upper respiratory tract infection. In a small number of cases, reparative surgery may be necessary.

TABLE 3.3—Indications for tracheostomy

- To relieve glottic or supraglottic obstruction
- To facilitate long term ventilatory support
- To facilitate continuous positive airway pressure (especially after chest injury)
- To facilitate speech through artificial airway, using special adaptors

Tracheostomy is necessary for patients requiring long term ventilation, long term airway protection, or tracheal suctioning.[16] Complications with intubation may also lead to the decision to use tracheostomy (table 3.3). Continuous positive airway pressure can be administered for long periods through a tracheostomy, or a facial mask. Once a tracheostomy has been provided it offers the chance of staged decannulation, using fenestrated tubes and tracheal buttons,[16] and this may permit an early transfer out of the intensive care unit.

A fixed policy, of tracheostomy after a set period of intubation, is becoming less popular.[17] Patients with facial injuries may require tracheostomy from the outset. Patients who will clearly require intubation for a long time, as in Guillain–Barré syndrome[18] and tetanus[19] should receive a tracheostomy as soon as possible. Patients with chest trauma requiring continuous positive airway pressure may be awake with regional analgesia, and find tracheostomy more tolerable than intubation. On the other hand, with improvements in tube design, and attention to risk factors for laryngeal damage, many feel that intubation may be tolerated for longer periods than was previously thought.[17]

Although the operating theatre provides the best surgical environment in which to perform tracheostomy, there are risks and costs associated with transferring patients out of the intensive care unit. It is possible to perform tracheostomy in the intensive care unit, provided equipment and trained assistance are available for the surgeon.[20–22] Percutaneous tracheostomy using needle, guide wire and serial dilators is now possible[23] and can be carried out under general anaesthesia by staff in the intensive care unit. However, because mid-line blood vessels can cause problems after inadequate blunt dissection, surgical assistance must always be immediately available. Minitracheostomy is useful for patients who are unable to expectorate, though they do not require continuous positive airway pressure or artificial ventilation. It is used as an adjunct to physiotherapy.[24] Such procedures can be carried out at

TABLE 3.4—Complications of tracheostomy

At insertion
- Incisional haemorrhage
- Pneumothorax, pneumomediastinum, subcutaneous emphysema

Early
- Stomal haemorrhage
- Aspiration of pharyngeal and gastric contents past a deflated cuff

Late
- Stomal infection
- Obstruction of lumen
- Swallowing dysfunction
- Erosion into oesophagus or innominate artery
- Abnormal scar or granuloma formation
- Tracheal stenosis at stoma or tip position
- Sepsis (bronchial or intrapulmonary)

---

the bedside, using local anaesthesia.[25] They carry many of the same risks as full tracheostomy.[21]

Early complications of tracheostomy include pneumothorax and pneumomediastinum, subcutaneous emphysema, incisional haemorrhage and tube displacement. Aspiration of gastric contents may occur during any airway manoeuvre where the protective reflexes are obtunded. The higher cricothyrotomy approach may produce laryngeal injury, but is not associated with pleural damage. Stomal bleeding is common, although usually not serious. Stomal infection is seen in about 12% of all tracheostomies,[22] and often arises 4 or 5 days after surgery (table 3.4).

Later complications of tracheostomy include tube obstruction, aspiration, swallowing dysfunction, and erosion into the oesophagus or the innominate artery. Even if stenosis does not occur, abnormal scar formation and granuloma may occur at the stoma site.[26] Tracheal stenosis only produces stridor in adults when over 75% of the lumen is obstructed.[27] Assessment of this injury is best done with lateral soft tissue radiographs of the neck, with fluoroscopy. Flow volume loops and CT scanning are less sensitive. The most direct assessment of tracheal stenosis is by fibreoptic bronchoscopy or fibreoptic laryngoscopy, though these procedures carry an anaesthetic risk.

All artificial airways require humidification or at least the conservation of exhaled water vapour. Heat and moisture exchangers are adequate for most cases, though high flow rates and tenacious

TABLE 3.5—Sedation scoring system*

- Fully alert
- Roused by voice
- Roused by pain
- Unrousable
- Paralysed
- Asleep

* Shelly MP, Dodds P, Park GR.[40]

secretions may demand a heated humidifier.[28] The use of bacteriostatic materials is now common.

Patients with tracheal tubes or tracheostomies are vulnerable to infection because of disrupted local clearance mechanisms, underlying immunosuppression, frequent suctioning, and the microbiological environment of the intensive care unit.[29] Viral infection is easily spread from staff to patient.[30] Contamination of the tracheal tube often precedes pneumonia by 2–4 days.[31] *Pseudomonas aeruginosa* is associated specifically with tracheostomy.[32]

Sedation and analgesia

Patients in the intensive care unit are exposed to many harmful or unpleasant stimuli. Some are later forgotten, but even temporarily unpleasant sensations should be avoided if possible. Among the common problems are anxiety, pain, lack of rest, thirst, and the use of the following: tracheal tube, face mask, nasogastric tube, physiotherapy, and urinary catheter.[33] Any nursing procedures, such as turning or changing dressings, are likely to be, at the least, uncomfortable.

The staff of the intensive care unit can alleviate many of these problems by careful explanation and appropriate reassurance.[34] Attitudes to the use of sedative drugs have changed[35 36] and there is increasing recognition that sedation, analgesia, and muscle relaxation should be provided specifically where indicated.[37-39] Muscle relaxants are neither sedative nor analgesic. Awareness of paralysis is both terrifying and avoidable and should be prevented by the use of sedatives.

Apart from subjective assessments of the adequacy of sedation, several sedation scoring systems have been designed. One system uses simple endpoints: fully alert; roused by voice; roused by pain; unrousable; paralysed; or asleep (table 3.5).[40] Another identifies

TABLE 3.6—The ideal sedative drug

- Rapid onset and recovery after bolus or infusion
- Wide therapeutic margin of safety
- Minimal cardiovascular effects
- Minimal and non-persistent respiratory depression
- Water solubility
- Absence of metabolic, immunological or hypersensitivity reactions
- Absence of confusion after cessation
- Low cost

anxiety or restlessness as a separate category.[41] In the future, auditory evoked potentials may be measured to determine the level of sedation in paralysed patients.[42] It is desirable that the same assessment approach is used by all staff in an intensive care unit so that comparative assessments can be made between patients and between drug therapy.

The simplest method of administering sedation and analgesia is by repeated bolus doses. This, however permits peaks and troughs of awareness and pain, which can be avoided using intravenous infusions.[33] The institution of an infusion should be preceded by a loading dose, taking account of any cardiovascular or respiratory depressant effects which the drug may have. The rectal route has also been used[43] and subcutaneous infusions of opiates can be effective. Patient controlled sedation and analgesia are also in use in some centres.[44]

The ideal sedative (and analgesic) drug has been described[45-47] as having the following properties: rapid onset and recovery by bolus or infusion; wide therapeutic index; minimal cardiovascular effects; respiratory depression which does not persist; water solubility; lack of irritation to veins; absence of metabolic, immunological or hypersensitivity reactions; and an absence of confusion after the drug is stopped. Such a drug should also be cheap (table 3.6). This is a tall order, and no drug approaches it. Many intensive care units use a combination of opiates and benzodiazepines, by bolus or infusion,[35] but there has never been a wholly satisfactory alternative to the effective but dangerous drugs, etomidate and althesin.[48]

Opiates are widely used, with each intensive care unit having current preferences. All pure opiate agonists are respiratory depressants and antitussives, which may be useful; however, these properties may delay weaning from the ventilator. Vasodilatation is common, which may be dangerous in the hypovolaemic patient. Gastric emptying and intestinal motility are slowed by opiates, and this can delay enteral feeding. Tolerance to analgesia is common, but addiction is very unlikely if the drug is used for a patient in pain.[49] It is inappropriate to rely on opiates alone for sedation, in view of their problems, especially in renal impairment, where their clearance may be very slow.[36 39]

Morphine is very useful (and cheap), but it has active metabolites. Papaveretum, being 50% morphine, has similar properties. One of its other constituents, noscapine, may be genotoxic[50]; this has lead to a rapid decline in its use. The short duration of action of a single bolus dose of fentanyl is due to redistribution rather than clearance, and its elimination half life is longer than that of morphine; there are therefore few indications for its use in intravenous infusions.[51]

Alfentanil[45 52–56] is purely analgesic. It is useful for awake patients and those shortly to be weaned from sedation. It has a short elimination half life and a small volume of distribution, and is well suited to continuous intravenous infusion. It is nevertheless dependent on hepatic metabolism and is expensive.

The use of regional analgesia is increasing, and the use of epidural opiates does not require such precise placement of the epidural catheter as do local anaesthetics. The risk from respiratory depression is much reduced in an intensive care unit, where constant monitoring and observation should forestall complications. Non-opioid analgesics may be given intramuscularly or rectally. Indomethacin can reduce opiate requirements, particularly post-operatively,[41] however, it may cause gastrointestinal bleeding.

The benzodiazepines are purely sedative, and when used alone their use is inappropriate for patients in pain. They also reduce muscle tone, and promote amnesia. Diazepam has an active metabolite (N-desmethyl diazepam) which has a long elimination half life, and this reduces its usefulness for intravenous infusion.

Midazolam is water soluble and has an elimination half life of 1–5 hours after prolonged infusion.[57] It is particularly useful for intravenous infusion, but bolus doses may produce hypotension, especially in the hypovolaemic patient.[58] It has a large volume of distribution in some patients, particularly in those with hypoalbuminaemia.[59 60] This may explain the apparently unpredictable prolonged effect in patients with multiple organ failure.[61] There is possibly a pharmacogenetic abnormality of midazolam clearance in 6–10% of the normal population.[62] Tolerance is sometimes observed during prolonged infusion.[63] Paediatric use of midazolam is common.[64 65] The use of flumazenil to provide temporary reversal of midazolam sedation has been recommended for neurological assessment,[66] though sedative agents with shorter half lives are available for this purpose.

Chlormethiazole given by intravenous infusion gives rapid onset sedation that is easily adjustable, and is specifically anticonvulsant,[67] but it contains a large water load, and is slow to wear off.[68]

Chloral hydrate is often given to neonates and infants nasogastrically, and reduces opiate and benzodiazepine requirements.

Chlorpromazine is useful given intramuscularly or rectally to calm patients suffering from opiate or other drug withdrawal. Its alpha blocking properties may cause problems in hypovolaemic patients.

Ketamine is unique as a sedative because it causes raised arterial resistance and bronchodilatation. These effects can be useful in either the hypovolaemic or asthmatic patient. Concurrent use of midazolam may reduce psychological after effects.[69]

Propofol infusions are increasingly used in the intensive care unit[46 70] The very short half life of this drug after prolonged infusion is a clear advantage. It can produce hypotension, especially in patients with hypovolaemia.[71] The combination of propofol and alfentanil,[72] while expensive, is well suited to patients with head injuries requiring regular assessment, and those withdrawing from longer acting sedative and analgesic agents. Propofol clearance is dependent on hepatic blood flow as much as metabolism.[73] Reports of persistent metabolic acidosis and myocardial failure in children receiving propofol infusions[74] have ruled out its use in paediatric intensive care.

Inhaled sedative agents, such as isoflurane, have been introduced in some intensive care units,[75-77] where scavenging of exhaled gas is possible. The cost of this use of isoflurane is great, which has discouraged its widespread use.[78] Reductions in plasma catecholamine levels are seen with this agent.[79] Plasma inorganic fluoride levels may rise to a peak days after the treatment is stopped[80 81]; the renal significance of this is not yet clear.

The pharmacological choices for sedation and analgesia in the intensive care unit are many, but in the end each unit tends to have its own policy, which medical and nursing staff clearly understand. This is a sensible approach, as long as alternatives are constantly considered.

Non-respiratory monitoring of the ventilated patient

Haemodynamic monitoring is essential when the critically ill patient is ventilated. All patients should have a correctly sited central venous pressure line. Central venous pressure measurements are useful in the fluid management of patients who have no appreciable pulmonary hypertension or cardiovascular disease. It is important for the patient not to have a low central venous pressure before assisted ventilation is started as the combination of an inadequate venous return to the right heart and positive pressure ventilation may lead to a catastrophic fall in blood pressure. The alterations in cardiac output during positive pressure ventilation have been ascribed to alterations in preload, with increased intrathoracic pressure causing peripheral translocation of central blood volume.[82] The elegant work of Wise et al[83 84] and Sylvester et al[85] has examined many of the factors affecting ventricular performance during mechanical ventilation with positive end expiratory pressure. It is now accepted that where ventilator reserve is limited and positive end expiratory pressure and ventilator settings have to be adjusted these adjustments should be made to optimise oxygen delivery and mixed venous oxygen saturation (which should if possible be over 70%). As with right atrial pressure, measurement of pulmonary capillary wedge pressure requires correct zero recordings and calibration; the measurement should be taken from the "a" wave at end expiration so that the level is not influenced by respiratory pressures.[86]

Other requirements for accurate measurement are enumerated in table 3.7. A pulmonary capillary wedge pressure below 18 mm Hg is not associated with pressure related pulmonary oedema but relates to oedema secondary to increased capillary permeability. Pressure related pulmonary oedema generally develops above pressures of 25 mm Hg, but in patients with longstanding high left atrial pressures oedema may not develop until the pulmonary capillary wedge pressure is over 30 mm Hg.

In patients with high airway pressures the difference between the pressure transmitted to the catheter tip (wedge pressure) and that transmitted to the left atrium cannot be predicted.[87] In critically ill patients the mean effective pulmonary capillary pressure

TABLE 3.7—Conditions for accurate measurement of pulmonary capillary wedge pressure in the ventilated patient

- Correct zero and calibration
- Measure at end expiration from the "a" wave
- Ensure that the catheter tip is sited below the level of the left atrium
- Ensure no interference with pulmonary venous drainage between the catheter tip and left atrium (for example pulmonary embolus)
- There should be no appreciable gradient between left atrium and left ventricle (for example mitral valve disease, where large "v" waves may be mistaken for "a" waves)
- When the balloon is deflated there should be a distinct pulmonary artery trace
- Should a wedge trace appear, the catheter must be withdrawn until the pulmonary artery trace reappears

(measured from the downstroke of the wedge pressure as the point when the rapid decline changes to a slower decline) may be a better measure than pulmonary capillary wedge pressure, as any increase in the former may worsen gas exchange.[88]

Cardiac output measurements are usually made by using a pulmonary artery catheter with a thermistor probe at its tip. The thermodilution technique is as accurate and reproducible as the dye dilution technique, provided that the catheter is placed accurately, the volume and temperature ($0°C$) of the injectate are accurate, and the injection is always performed at the same point in the respiratory cycle. The derived variable, oxygen delivery, is of particular value for optimising ventilation and can be combined with the measurement of mixed venous oxygen saturation ($S\bar{v}o_2$) in the pulmonary artery, by blood sampling or the use of a catheter with an optical probe at its tip. Mixed venous oxygen saturation may not be an early predictor of change in cardiac output but it provides an indication of the delicate balance between oxygen delivery and extraction. Dual oximetry (simultaneous monitoring of (Sao_2 and $S\bar{v}o_2$) Sao_2) and mixed is of considerable value when adjusting ventilatory indices during ventilation, giving a continuous visual guide of the effects of alteration without recourse to blood gas analysis. Dual oximetry can also be used for assessment of venous admixture (Qsp/Qt).[89] Provided pulmonary end capillary blood can be assumed to be fully saturated with oxygen a ventilation–perfusion index (VQI), can be derived from the formula used for calculating Qsp/Qt.

$$Qsp/Qt = 100 \cdot (1 - Sao_2)(1 - S\bar{v}o_2) = VQI$$

$S\bar{v}o_2$ should be standardised daily by co-oximetry.

TABLE 3.8—Indications for measuring cardiac output, oxygen delivery, and mixed venous oxygen saturation in the ventilated patient

- Raised central venous pressure
- Appearance of pulmonary oedema on the chest radiograph
- Hypotension in the presence of normal central venous pressure and hypervolaemic response to volume challenge
- Optimisation of ventilation
- Optimisation of inotropic support

Indications for haemodynamic monitoring and measurement of derived variables are listed in table 3.8. Recent work has explained the importance of right ventricular performance in patients with acute respiratory failure[90] and how it changes with positive end expiratory pressure. Measurement of right ventricular volume variables has been made possible by the "fast response" thermodilution technique. Bronet and coworkers[90] found that, though in many patients with acute respiratory failure and increasing pulmonary hypertension the right ventricle dilated and right ventricular ejection fraction decreased, stroke volume was maintained unless there was concomitant disease, such as septic shock or viral myocarditis. Preload augmentation in these patients is clearly important, and it is necessary in respiratory failure to ensure that left atrial pressures are maintained. Positive end expiratory pressure has been found to have two effects on right ventricular function.[91] In most patients it causes unloading of the right ventricle by reducing venous return, and in a few it leads to right ventricular dilatation and a decreased ejection fraction. A further study suggested that the changes in the right ventricle induced by positive end expiratory pressure are probably a function of the initial right ventricular ejection fraction and right ventricular end diastolic volume index.[92]

Nutrition in the ventilated patient

Acute weight loss of 30–40% of the original body weight is usually lethal,[93] and maximal physical performance is impaired in healthy individuals who have lost around 10% of body weight.[94] Increased mortality and morbidity correlate closely with an acute loss of 10–30% of the individual's normal body weight.[95]

Clearly the best route for providing nutrition is the gastrointestinal tract. Calories given via the gastrointestinal tract maintain the integrity of the liver and oxidation of nutrients, a process that

TABLE 3.9—Check list before feeding

- All electrolyte deficiencies must be corrected
- Acid–base state must be stable
- Adjust ventilation to ensure a normal arterial oxygen tension
- Ensure normal calcium, magnesium, and inorganic phosphate concentrations
- Determine serum B_{12}, folate, and albumin concentrations before starting treatment
- Cardiac and renal function must be known
- Tolerance to a glucose load must be known
- Is there evidence of hepatocellular failure?

---

is imprecisely understood.[96] Enteral feeding rarely produces the hepatic parenchymal changes seen with intravenous feeding.[97] Animal studies have shown that normal gastrointestinal morphology is better maintained by enteral feeding.[98] This route is often not suitable, however, in the ventilated patient because of the nature of the illness and the use of drugs that suppress bowel motility. When bowel absorption is not possible intravenous nutrition may be necessary, but it is important to reintroduce gastrointestinal feeding as soon as possible. When it is reintroduced after several days or weeks of parenteral nutrition, it must be done gradually; diarrhoea may ensue unless the osmolality of the feed is increased slowly over several days.

In the critically ill ventilated patient, metabolic and volume normality must be established before nutrition is started (table 3. 9). When a normal arterial carbon dioxide tension cannot be achieved by adjusting the ventilator settings, the total calories given as glucose should be reduced to cut down carbon dioxide production.

Parenteral nutrition should be given via a designated feeding line. The line is best tunnelled subcutaneously and is generally inserted into the subclavian vein by the infraclavicular technique. This method may be complicated in the ventilated patient by a pneumothorax, and should therefore be avoided in patients with poor respiratory function (low arterial oxygen tension and saturation despite optimum ventilation and high fractional inspired oxygen), particularly when airway pressures are high. In these circumstances a feeding line may be inserted high into the internal jugular vein and tunnelled in the neck.

Energy requirements for critically ill patients have traditionally been established by the use of the Harris–Benedict equation.[99] The

TABLE 3.10—Determination of energy requirements for total parenteral nutrition*

Formula for estimating energy requirements:
Normal (1) basal metabolic rate × "stress factor" (2) × 1·25 (3) = daily energy requirement for weight maintenance + 1000 (4) kcal – daily energy requirement for weight gain

1 *Normal basal metabolic rate* can be determined by using standard nomograms or formulas (usually 1500–1800 kcal/day).
Approximate resting metabolic rates for adults of average size

Body weight (kg)	50	55	60	65	70	80
kcal/day	1316	1411	1509	1602	1694	1872

2 *"Stress factor"*: the normal basal metabolic weight corrected for the disease process stress factor applied to the normal basal metabolic rate.

Mild starvation	0·85–1·00
Postoperative (no complication)	1·00–1·05
Cancer†	1·10–1·45
Peritonitis†	1·05–1·25
Severe infection or multiple trauma†	1·30–1·55
Burn†	1·50–1·70

3 The basal caloric requirements of stressed patients are not adjusted upward when they are heavily sedated and ventilated, but consider an increase of up to 20% in non-sedated patients.

4 If anabolism and weight gain are the goals, an additional 1000 calories/day may be added.

---

* Modified from Apelgren and Wilmore.[100]
† Proportional to the extent of disease or injury.
Conversion from traditional to SI units: 1 kcal = 4·184 kJ.

total energy expenditure is then calculated by multiplying the basal metabolic rate by a stress factor, which may be augmented by an allowance for physical activity. This method was admirably described by Apelgren and Wilmore,[100] and is still being used in units where the total energy expenditure cannot be estimated by indirect calorimetry (table 3.10). Cortes and Nelson[101] showed that clinical assessment may overestimate energy expenditure because the apparent degree of illness used as the basis for determining the stress factor is not an accurate guide. Not only is bedside calorimetry useful in assessing energy expenditure more accurately but it may also lead to financial saving. Liggett and Renfro[102] described an alternative method for estimating energy expenditure based on the assumption that the respiratory quotient is 0·85. They claim this incurs a small error of $\pm 3\%$. Carbohydrate has a respiratory quotient of 1, fat 0·7, and protein 0·82. However, during lipogenesis (synthesis of fat from glucose) the quotient rises to 8. The method requires measurement of cardiac output, $S\bar{v}o_2$, Sao_2, and haemoglobin concentration, and when fixed constants are combined and appropriate unit conversions performed, the equation provides energy expenditure expressed as kcal/day. Liggett and Renfro[102] studied 73 mechanically ventilated non-surgical patients with various types of critical illness, and concluded that calorific requirements in this group can be estimated by the use of the Harris–Benedict equation without extensive modifications, but that an increase of 20% above these calculated levels was necessary in septic patients.

In respiratory failure, adjustment of the ventilator settings to lower the arterial carbon dioxide tension may not be possible. In these circumstances, to avoid hypermetabolism related to a high glucose load, the proportion of carbohydrate non-nitrogen containing calories should be 40–60%, the rest being given as fat.[103]

The use of fat rather than dextrose as a source of calories has two advantages. The respiratory quotient of fat oxidation is 0·7, compared with 1·0 for dextrose, so carbon dioxide production is lower; and fat, being iso-osmolar and of neutral pH, can be given via a peripheral vein.

Protein both increases protein synthesis and diminishes the rate of catabolism. Whereas non-protein calories may improve nitrogen balance in mild to moderately catabolic individuals, protein alone (at a rate of 1·5–2·0 g/kg/day) may be sufficient to preserve lean body mass.[104 105] Considerable attention should therefore be focused on the nature and quantity of protein administered. Many critically ill patients retain less protein than is administered, and for this reason branched chain amino acid enriched formulas have been developed in the hope of improving nitrogen retention. Investigations so far have not found these formulas are of benefit. Branched chain amino acids depleted of aromatic amino acids have been suggested as a valuable protein source in hepatic encephalopathy. However, investigations suggest that the usual formulations can be given safely to patients who are encephalopathic.[106] The majority of critically ill patients require at least 1·5 g/kg/day of protein to achieve nitrogen equilibrium.

Nitrogen requirements are generally assessed by measuring the urinary urea nitrogen lost in the urine.[107]

Nitrogen (N) balance = grams of N–grams of urea N + 4 g
$$\quad\quad\quad\quad\quad\quad\quad\text{IN}\quad\quad\quad\quad\text{OUT}$$

The 4 g factor accounts for the unmeasured nitrogen losses in skin and stool. Askanazi and coworkers[108] investigated the respiratory response of patients to increasing protein supply and found that progressive increase enhanced ventilatory drive and minute volume. In patients with limited reserve, however, this may lead to respiratory failure in the spontaneously breathing patient. Precise protein requirements in patients requiring ventilatory support remain to be established.[108] Even in the presence of high nitrogen losses the nitrogen load is rarely increased above 14 g/day.

It is important in parenteral feeding to assess electrolyte and fluid balance regularly, giving special attention to potassium and phosphate requirements. Hypophosphataemia is known to reduce oxygen transport and energy supply and when severe may lead to respiratory failure.[109] Vitamins and trace elements should be replaced if feeding is continued for more than 5 days. Shenkin[110] has recently stressed the difficulty of assessing trace element states in seriously ill patients and in establishing the amount of trace element supplements to provide during nutritional support. Prolonged nutrition is best supplied by a mixture of protein, fat, electrolytes, vitamins, and trace elements made up into a 3 litre bag, prescribed early in the morning and supplied by the pharmacy later in the day. The mixture has to be carefully compiled to ensure compatibility between the different constituents of the feed.

Some studies suggest that ventilator weaning may be facilitated by preceding nutritional support.[111][112] Evidence suggests that respiratory muscle function is diminished in poorly nourished patients. Kelly[113] evaluated initial maximum inspiratory mouth pressure as an index of respiratory muscle function in 51 patients in hospital. Malnourished patients were found to have significantly less inspiratory force than normally nourished patients. The electrolyte content of the diet is particularly important during weaning (table 3.11). Further details on nutrition are supplied by Apelgren and Wilmore,[100] and, for acute respiratory failure, by Pingleton.[114] McMahon and co-workers[115] give a fascinating review of the

TABLE 3.11—Nutritional considerations during weaning

- Observe arterial carbon dioxide tension in relation to carbohydrate load
- Ensure a non-protein calorie:nitrogen ratio of around 150:1
- Carbohydrate load should be 40–60% of total non-protein calories, the rest being given as fat
- Nitrogen load should in general not exceed 14 g daily; if hyperventilation is present consider the possibility that the nitrogen load is excessive
- Ensure a normal serum phosphate and potassium content
- Observe the fluid balance; do *not* overload

importance of basic established concepts of exercise physiology and nutritional support applied to weaning from mechanical ventilation.

Psychological and sleep disturbances during assisted ventilation

Psychiatric symptoms relating to assisted ventilation will not be manifest while the patient is heavily sedated and ventilation is controlled but are likely to emerge during weaning. It is clearly important to exclude organic dysfunction of the brain and physiological derangements due to blood gas or metabolic abnormalities.

The intensive care environment is recognised to cause stress, as a result of the alien and frightening atmosphere, sleep deprivation, unfamiliar noise, and a feeling of being confined by equipment.[116] Assisted ventilation produces additional stresses, related to awareness of the endotracheal or tracheostomy tube, the discomfort of suction and complicating hypoxia, and the horror of depending on a machine for ventilation.

Gries and Fernsler[117] conducted a survey to assess the causes of stress associated with ventilation in 17 patients, whose ages ranged from 35 to 81 years. Five patients could not recall the period of ventilation and three did not wish to discuss the problem. The others categorised the stresses as shown in table 3.12. The major complaints were related to restriction of activity, the awareness and unpleasantness of the tracheal tube, suction, and the process of extubation. Inability to communicate was also frustrating. Some had vivid dreams, probably related to drugs. The more serious psychological problems (the intensive care syndrome) include disturbances of cognitive, affective, and perceptual functions. These occur in 12·5–18% of patients,[118–121] and are likely to be related to metabolic, neurological, or pharmacological factors. Many are

49

TABLE 3.12—Stressors associated with mechanical ventilation*

Intrapersonal: physiological
Frustration from activity restriction
Awareness of spontaneous breathing restriction related to ventilation

Intrapersonal: psychosocial and cultural
Insufficient explanation and hence misinterpretation of medical condition
Activity restriction producing a feeling of inability to cope
Ventilator dependence
Vivid dreams
Awareness of extubation

Interpersonal
Insufficient explanations
Inability to communicate
Loss of confidence in and criticism of nursing care

Extrapersonal
Unpleasant experiences relating to
• the tracheal tube
• suctioning
• extubation
• noise (from ventilator or surroundings)

---

* Modified from Gries and Fernsler.[117]

related to drug dependence and withdrawal, and commonly occur during weaning. Hallucinations (pleasant and unpleasant) are common, and may manifest themselves as aggression, non-recognition of relatives, periods of agitation, and non-cooperation. These changes are most likely to arise in the patient who has been ventilated for a long time or who has previously been dependent on drugs, for example benzodiazepines, opiates, or alcohol. Drug withdrawal during weaning from the ventilator may be extremely difficult. Methadone is useful, enabling opiates to be rapidly reduced, and on occasion, where they are considered safe, beta blocking drugs may alleviate the tachycardia and anxiety related to opiate withdrawal. Rectal chlorpromazine given regularly, at the onset of weaning, has a potent calming effect without depressing the respiratory centre.

Gale and O'Shanick[122] discussed preventive psychological interactions for the ventilated patient, which are noted, with modifications, in table 3.13. Communication problems may in the future be reduced by the use of a word processor by the patient.[123]

Patients in an intensive care unit rarely sleep for more than a few hours at a time,[124] and frequently do not complete a sleep

TABLE 3.13—Preventive psychological interactions

Communication problems
Talk to the patient
Provide alphabet, sign, or picture board, writing tablet or word processor

Dependence and loss of control
Allow the patient choice when possible (position in bed, radio station)
Keep patient informed of progress
Inform patient of procedures to be undertaken, and the reasons for them

Fear of death or disability
Explain the ventilator and its alarm systems
Inform the patient of changes in ventilator settings and the reasons for them
Allow the patient to express any emotional problems and give support
Keep discussion and controversies about management away from the bedside

Isolation and fear of strangers
Establish continuity of care
Encourage visits by family and close friends

Sensory alteration
Maintain the patient's orientation with a calendar and clock on the wall, family photographs, and visits by relatives and close friends
Establish a day–night routine if at all possible
At night
● minimise noise
● minimise movement of and interference with the patient
● ensure adequate analgesia and maximise comfort
During the day provide a daytime environment with, for example, visits, television, music.

---

cycle. Completion of a sleep cycle is essential for maintaining and restoring physical and psychological functions. Experiments in which people are deprived of sleep show that after 2–5 days subjects become anxious, suspicious, and disorientated, some developing delusions and paranoia.[125] Lack of prolonged sleep may be an important factor contributing to the intensive care syndrome.[126] Weissman and colleagues[127] found that the average length of a sleep period in an intensive care unit was only 24 minutes. The noise level in an intensive care unit is high, and has been found to be a major cause of sleep deprivation.[128 129] Methods whereby a normal sleep cycle can be encouraged are summarised in table 3.13.

The psychological needs of the ventilated patient have so far received scant attention. Aspects of care include maintaining a normal sleep cycle, minimising noise (particularly at night), awareness of the problems associated with drug dependence and withdrawal, helping and communicating with patients, and endeavouring to establish reorientation and a pleasant and calm environment during weaning.

1 Brunel W, Coleman DL, Schwartz DE, Peper E, Cohen NH. Assessment of routine chest roentgenograms and the physical examination to confirm endotracheal tube position. *Chest* 1989;**96**:1043–5.
2 Astrachan DI, Kirchner JC, Goodwin WJ Jr. Prolonged intubation vs. tracheostomy: complications, practical and psychological considerations. *Laryngoscope* 1988;**98**:1165–9.
3 Scott PH, Eigen H, Moye LA, Georgitis J, Laughlin JJ. Predictability and consequences of spontaneous extubation in a paediatric ICU. *Crit Care Med* 1985;**13**:228–32.
4 Aebert H, Hunefeld G, Regel G. Paranasal sinusitis and sepsis in ICU patients with nasotracheal intubation. *Intensive Care Med* 1988;**1**:868–9.
5 Meyer P, Guerin JM, Habib Y, Levy C. Pseudomonas thoracic empyema secondary to nosocomial rhinosinusitis. *Eur Respir J* 1988;**102**:746–51.
6 Grindlinger GA, Niehoff J, Hughes SL, Humphrey MA, Simpson G. Acute paranasal sinusitis related to nasotracheal intubation of head-injured patients. *Crit Care Med* 1987;**15**:214–7.
7 Kronberg FG, Goodwin WJ Jr. Sinusitis in intensive care unit patients. *Laryngoscope* 1985;**95**:936–8.
8 Pippin LK, Short DH, Bowes JB. Long-term tracheal intubation practice in the United Kingdom. *Anaesthesia* 1983;**38**:791–5.
9 Chalon J, Ramanathan S. Care of the airway. *Int Anaesthesiol Clin* 1986;**24**:53–64.
10 Kastanos N, Estopa-Miro R, Marin-Perez A, Xaubert-Mir A, Agusti-Vidal A. Laryngotracheal injury due to endotracheal intubation: incidence, evolution, and predisposing factors. A prospective long-term study. *Crit Care Med* 1983;**11**:362–7.
11 Marsh HM, Gillespie DJ, Baumgartner AE. Timing of tracheostomy in the critically ill patient. *Chest* 1989;**96**:190–3.
12 Loubser MD, Mahoney PJ, Milligan DW. Hazards of routine endotracheal suction in the neonatal unit. *Lancet* 1989;**1**:1444–5.
13 Bailey C, Kattwinkel J, Teja K, Buckley T. Shallow versus deep endotracheal suctioning in young rabbits: pathologic effects on the tracheobronchial wall. *Paediatrics* 1988;**98**:1165–9.
14 Dankle SK, Schuller DE, McClead RE. Prolonged intubation of neonates. *Arch Otolaryngol Head Neck Surg* 1987;**113**:841–3.
15 Jones R, Bodnar A, Roan Y, Johnson D. Subglottic stenosis in newborn intensive care unit graduates. *Am J Dis Child* 1981;**135**:367–8.
16 Stock MC, Woodward CG, Shapiro BA, Cane RD, Lewis V, Pecaro B. Perioperative complications of elective tracheostomy in critically ill patients. *Crit Care Med* 1986;**14**:861–3.
17 Watson CB. A survey of intubation practices in critical care medicine. *Ear Nose Throat J* 1983;**62**:494–501.
18 Gracey DR, McMichan JC, Divertie MB, Howard FM Jr. Respiratory failure in Guillain–Barré syndrome: a 6-year experience. *Mayo Clin Proc* 1982;**57**:742–6.
19 Udwardia FE, Lall A, Udwardia ZF, Sekhar M, Vora A. Tetanus and its complications: intensive care and management experience in 150 Indian patients. *Epidemiol Infect* 1987;**99**:675–84.
20 Hawkins ML, Burrus EP, Treat RC, Mansberger AR Jr. Tracheostomy in the intensive care unit: a safe alternative to the operating room. *South Med J* 1989;**82**:1096–8.
21 Stevens DJ, Howard DJ. Tracheostomy service for ITU patients. *Ann R Coll Surg Engl* 1988;**70**:241–2.
22 Dayal VS, el Masri W. Tracheostomy in intensive care setting. *Laryngoscope* 1986;**96**:58–60.
23 Bodenham A, Diament R, Cohen A, Webster N. Percutaneous dilational tracheostomy. A bedside procedure on the Intensive Care Unit. *Anaesthesia* 1991;**46**:570–2.
24 Lewis GA, Hopkinson RB, Matthews HR. Minitracheotomy. A report on its use in intensive therapy. *Anaesthesia* 1986;**41**:931–5.
25 Hazard PB, Garrett HE Jr, Adams JW, Robbins ET, Aguillard RN. Bedside percutaneous tracheostomy: experience with 55 elective procedures. *Ann Thorac Surg* 1988;**46**:63–7.

26 Schloss MD, Gold JA, Rosales JK, Baxter JD. Acute epiglottitis: current management. *Laryngoscope* 1983;**93**:489–93.
27 Heffner JE, Miller KS, Sahn SA. Tracheostomy in the intensive care unit. Part 2: Complications. *Chest* 1986;**90**:430–6.
28 Cohen IL, Weinberg PF, Fein IA, Rowinski GS. Endotracheal tube occlusion associated with the use of heat and moisture exchangers in the intensive care unit. *Crit Care Med* 1988;**16**:277–9.
29 Salata RA, Lederman MM, Shlaes DM *et al*. Diagnosis of nosocomial pneumonia in intubated, intensive care unit patients. *Am Rev Respir Dis* 1987;**135**:426–32.
30 Valenti WM, Clarke TA, Hall CB, Menegus MA, Shapiro DL. Concurrent outbreaks of rhinovirus and respiratory syncitial virus in an intensive care nursery: epidemiology and associated risk factors. *J Paediatr* 1982;**100**:722–6.
31 Comhaire A, Lamy M. Contamination rate of sterilized ventilators in an ICU. *Crit Care Med* 1981;**9**:546–8.
32 Freeman R, McPeake PK. Acquisition, spread, and control of *Pseudomonas aeruginosa* in a cardiothoracic intensive care unit. *Thorax* 1982;**37**:732–6.
33 Aitkenhead AR. Analgesia and sedation in intensive care. *Br J Anaesth* 1989;**63**:196–206.
34 Sedation in the intensive care unit (editorial). *Lancet* 1984;**1**:1388–9.
35 Bion JF, Ledingham IM. Sedation in intensive care – a postal survey. *Intensive Care Med* 1987;**13**:215–6.
36 Gast PH, Fisher A, Sear JW. Intensive care sedation now. *Lancet* 1984;**2**:863–4.
37 Miller-Jones CM, Williams JH. Sedation for ventilation. A retrospective study of 50 patients. *Anaesthesia* 1980;**35**:1104–6.
38 Edbrooke DM, Hebron BS, Mather SJ, Dixon AM. Etomidate infusion: a method of sedation for the intensive care unit. *Anaesthesia* 1981;**36**:65.
39 Aitkenhead AR, Pepperman ML, Willatts SM, *et al*. Comparison of propofol and midazolam for sedation in critically ill patients. *Lancet* 1989;**2**:704–9.
40 Shelly MP, Dodds P, Park GR. Assessing sedation. *Care of the Critically Ill* 1986;**2**:170–1.
41 Ramsay MAE, Savage TM, Simpson BRJ, Goodwin R. Controlled sedation with alphaxalone/alphadolone. *Br Med J* 1974;**2**:656–9.
42 Sneyd JR, Wang DY, Edwards D, *et al*. Effect of physiotherapy on the auditory evoked response of paralysed, sedated patients in the intensive therapy unit. *Br J Anaesth* 1992;**68**:349–51.
43 Reasbeck PG, Rice ML, Reasbeck JC. Double blind controlled trial of indomethacin as an adjunct to narcotic analgesia after major abdominal surgery. *Lancet* 1982;**2**:115–8.
44 Loper KA, Ready LB, Brody M. Patient-controlled anxiolysis with midazolam. *Anaesth Analg* 1988;**67**:1118–9.
45 Yate PM, Thomas D, Short SM, Sebel PS, Morton J. Comparison of infusions of alfentanil or pethidine for sedation of ventilated patients on the ITU. *Br J Anaesth* 1988;**6**:583–8.
46 Beller JP, Pottecher T, Lugnier A, Mangin P, Otteni JC. Prolonged sedation with propofol in ICU patients: recovery and blood concentration changes during periodic interruptions in infusion. *Br J Anaesth* 1988;**61**:583–8.
47 Sear JW. Overview of drugs available for ITU sedation. *Eur J Anaesthesiol Suppl* 1987;**1**:55–61.
48 Ledingham IM, Bion JF, Newman LH, McDonald JC, Wallace PG. Mortality, and morbidity amongst sedated intensive care patients. *Resuscitation* 1988;**16**(Suppl):S69–77.
49 Merriman HM, The techniques used to sedate ventilated patients: a survey of methods used in 34 ICUs in Great Britain. *Intensive Care Medicine* 1981;**7**:217–24.
50 Committee on Safety of Medicines. Genotoxicity of papaveretum and noscapine. *Current Problems* 1991;No:30.
51 Shafer A, White PF, Schuttler J, Rosenthal MH. Use of a fentanyl infusion in the intensive care unit: tolerance to its anaesthetic effects? *Anesthesiology* 1983;**59**:245–8.
52 Cohen AT, Kelly DR. Assessment of alfentanil by intravenous infusion as long-term sedation in intensive care. *Anaesthesia* 1987;**42**:545–8.
53 Sear JE, Fisher A, Summerfield RJ. Is alfentanil by infusion useful for sedation on the ITU? *Eur J Anaesthesiol Suppl* 1987;**1**:63–6.
54 Cohen AT. Experience with alfentanil infusion as an intensive care sedative analgesic. *Eur J Anaesthesiol Suppl* 1987;**1**:67–70.
55 Sinclair ME, Sear JW, Summerfield RJ, Fisher A. Alfentanil infusions on the intensive therapy unit. *Intensive Care Med* 1988;**14**:55–9.

56 Yate PM, Thomas D, Sebel PS. Alfentanil infusion for sedation and analgesia in intensive care. *Lancet* 1984;2:396–7.
57 Klotz U, Reimann IW. Chronopharmacokinetic study with prolonged infusion of midazolam. *Clin Pharmacokinetics* 1984;9:469–74.
58 Geller E, Halpern P, Barzelai E, *et al.* Midazolam infusion and the benzodiazepine anatagonist flumazenil for sedation of intensive care patients. *Resuscitation* 1988;16(Suppl):S31–9.
59 Shelly MP, Mendel L, Park GR. Failure of critically ill patients to metabolise midazolam. *Anaesthesia* 1987;42:619–26.
60 Vree TB, Shimoda M, Driessen JJ, *et al.* Decreased plasma albumin concentration results in increased volume of distribution and decreased elimination of midazolam in intensive care patients. *Clin Pharmacol Ther* 1989;46:537–44.
61 Bodenham A, Park GR. Reversal of prolonged sedation using flumazenil in critically ill patients. *Anaesthesia* 1989;44:603–5.
62 Dundee JW, Collier PS, Carlisle RJ, Harper KW. Prolonged midazolam elimination half-life. *Br Clin Pharm* 1986;21:425 9.
63 Shelly MP, Sultan MA, Bodenham A, Park GR. Midazolam infusions in critically ill patients. *Eur J Anaesthesiol* 1991;8:21–7.
64 Silvasi DL, Rosen DA, Rosen KR. Continuous intravenous midazolam infusion for sedation in the paediatric intensive care unit. *Anesth Analg* 1988;67:286–8.
65 Shapiro JM, Westphal LM, White PF, Sladen RN, Rosenthal MH. Midazolam infusion for sedation in the intensive care unit: effect on adrenal function. *Anaesthesiology* 1986;64:394–8.
66 Fisher GC, Clapham MC, Hutton P. Flumazenil in intensive care. The duration of arousal after an assessment dose. *Anaesthesia* 1991;46:413–6.
67 Scott DB. Chlormethiazole in intensive care. *Acta Psychiatr Scand* 1986;329(Suppl):185–8.
68 Scott DB, Beamish D, Hudson IN, Jostell KG. Prolonged infusion of chlormethiazole in intensive care. *Br J Anaesth* 1980;52:541–5.
69 Park GR, Manara AR, Mendel L, Bateman PE. Ketamine infusion. Its use as a sedative, inotrope and bronchodilator in a critically ill patient. *Anaesthesia* 1987;42:980–3.
70 Farling PA, Johnston JR, Coppel DL. Propofol infusion for sedation of patients with head injury in intensive care. A preliminary report. *Anaesthesia* 1989;44:222–6.
71 Harris CE, Grounds RM, Murray AM, *et al.* Propofol for long-term sedation in the intensive care unit. A comparison with papaveretum and midazolam. *Anaesthesia* 1990;45:366–72.
72 Harper SJ, Buckley PM, Carr K. Propofol and alfentanil infusions for sedation in intensive therapy. *Eur J Anaesthesiol* 1991;8:157–65.
73 Bailie GR, Cockshott ID, Douglas EJ, Bowles BJ. Pharmacokinetics of propofol during and after long-term continuous infusion for maintenance of sedation in ICU patients. *Br J Anaesth* 1992;68:486–91.
74 Parke TJ, Stevens JE, Rice AS, *et al.* Metabolic acidosis and fatal myocardial failure after propofol infusion in children; five case reports. *Br Med J* 1992;305:613–6.
75 Beechey AP, Hull JM, McLellan I, Atherley DW. Sedation with isoflurane. *Anaesthesia* 1988;43;419–20.
76 Kong KL, Willatts SM, Prys-Roberts C. Isoflurane compared with midazolam for sedation in the intensive care unit. *Br Med J* 1989;298:1277–80.
77 Millane TA, Bennett ED, Grounds RM. Isoflurane and propofol for long-term sedation in the intensive care unit. A crossover study. *Anaesthesia* 1992;47:768–74.
78 Park GR, Burns AM. Isoflurane compared with midazolam in the intensive care unit. *Br Med J* 1989;298:1642.
79 Kong KL, Willatts SM, Prys-Roberts C, Harvey JT, Gorman S. Plasma catecholamine concentration during sedation in ventilated patients requiring intensive therapy. *Intensive Care Med* 1990;16:171–4.
80 Spencer EM, Willatts SM, Prys-Roberts C. Plasma inorganic fluoride concentrations during and after prolonged (>24 h) isoflurane sedation: effect on renal function. *Anaesthesia Analgesia* 1991;73:731–7.
81 Breheny FX. Inorganic fluoride in prolonged isoflurane sedation. *Anaesthesia* 1992;47:32–3.
82 Seely RD. Dynamic effect of inspiration on the stroke volume of the right and left ventricles. *Am J Physiol* 1980;154:273–80.
83 Wise R, Robotham J, Bromberger-Barnes B, Permutt S. The effect of PEEP on left ventricular function in right heart bypassed dogs. *J Appl Physiol* 1981;51:541–6.

84 Wise R, Robotham J, Bromberger-Barnes B, et al. Elevation of left ventricle diastolic pressure by PEEP in the isolated in-situ heart. Physiologist 1979;22:134–8.
85 Sylvester JT, Goldberg HS, Permautt S. The role of the vasculature in the regulation of cardiac output. Clin Chest Med 1983;4:111–26.
86 Runciman WB, Putten AJ, Ilsley AH. An evaluation of blood pressure measurement. Anaesth Intens Care 1981;9:314–25.
87 Downs JB, Douglas ME. Assessment of cardiac filling pressure during continuous positive pressure ventilation. Crit Care Med 1980;8:285–90.
88 Cope DK, Allison RC, Parmentier JL, Miller JN, Taylor AE. Measurement of effective pulmonary capillary pressure profile after pulmonary artery occlusion. Crit Care Med 1986;14:16–22.
89 Rasanen J, Downs JB, deHaven B. Titration of continuous positive airway pressure by real-time dual oximetry. Chest 1987;92:853–6.
90 Bronet F, Dhainaut JF, Devaux JY, Huyghebaert MF, Villemert D, Monsallier JF. Right ventricular performance in patients with acute respiratory failure. Intens Care Med 1988; 14:474–7.
91 Neidhert PP, Suter PM. Changes of right ventricular function with positive end expiratory pressure (PEEP) in man. Intens Care Med 1988;14:471–3.
92 Brienza A, Dambrosio M, Bruno F, Marucci M, Belpiede G, Giuliani R. Right ventricular ejection fraction. Measurement in acute respiratory failure (ARF). Effects of PEEP. Intens Care Med 1988;14:478–82.
93 Moore FD. Metabolic care of the surgical patient. Philadelphia: Saunders. 1959:421.
94 Keys A, Brozek J, Henschel A, et al. The biology of human starvation. Vol 1. Minneapolis: University of Minnesota Press, 1950:714.
95 Studley HO. Percentage of weight loss. A basic indicator of surgical risk in patients with chronic peptic ulcer. JAMA. 1936;106:458.
96 Defronzo RA, Jacot E, Jequier E, Maeder E, Wahren J, Felber JP. The effect of insulin on the disposal of intravenous glucose. Diabetes 1981;30:1000.
97 Schlichtig R, Cole Sargent S. Nutritional support of the mechanically ventilated patient. Crit Care Clin 1990;6:767–84.
98 Schlichtig R, Ayres SM. Modes of delivery: Rationale, implementation, and mechanical complications. In: Nutritional support of the critically ill. Chicago. Year Book Medical Publishers, 1988.
99 Harris JA, Benedict FG. A biometric study of basal metabolism in men. Washington DC: Carnegie Institute, publication No 279:1919.
100 Apelgren KN, Wilmore DW. Nutritional care of the critically ill patient. Surg Clin N Am 1983;63:487–507.
101 Cortes V, Nelson LD. Errors in estimating energy expenditure in critically ill surgical patients. Arch Surg 1989;124:287–90.
102 Liggett SB, Renfro AD. Energy expenditures of mechanically ventilated non-surgical patients. Clinical investigations in critical care. Chest 1990;98:682–6.
103 Askanazi J, Nordenstrom J, Rosenbaum SH, et al. Nutrition for the patient with respiratory failure. Glucose vs fat. Anaesthesiology 1981;54:373–7.
104 Humberstone DA, Koen J, Shaw, JHF. Relative importance of aminoacid infusion as a means of sparing protein in surgical patients. J Parent Enteral Nutr 1989;13:223–7.
105 Shizgal HM, Milne CA, Spanier AH. The effect of nitrogen sparing intravenously administered fluids on post-operative body composition. Surgery 1979;85:496–506.
106 Schlichtig R, Ayres SM. Nutritional considerations for specific disease states. In: Nutritional support of the critically ill. Chicago: Year Book Medical Publishers, 1988:185.
107 Barrett TA, Robin AP, Armstrong MK, et al. Nutrition and respiratory failure. In: Bone RC, George RB, Hudston LD, eds Acute respiratory failure. New York: Churchill Livingstone, 1987:265–303.
108 Askanazi J, Weissman C, Lafala PA, Milic-Emili J, Kinney JM. Effect of protein intake on ventilatory drive. Anaesthesiology 1984;60:106–10.
109 Spector N. Nutritional support of the ventilator dependent patient. Nursing Clin North Am 1989;24:407–14.
110 Shenkin A. Trace elements and acute illness. Care of the Critically Ill 1993;9:60–3.
111 Larca L, Greenbaum DM. Effectiveness of intensive nutritional regimens in patients who fail to wean from mechanical ventilation. Crit Care Med 1982;10:297–300.
112 Bassili HR, Deitel M. Effect of nutritional support on weaning patients off mechanical ventilation. J Parenter Enteral Nutr 1981;5:161–3.

113 Kelly SM, Rosa A, Field S, Coughlin N, Schizgal HM, Macklem PT. Inspiratory muscle strength and body composition in patients receiving parenteral nutrition therapy. *Am Rev Respir Dis* 1984;**130**:33–7.
114 Pingleton SK. Nutrition in acute respiratory failure. *Lung* 1986;**164**:127–37.
115 McMahon MM, Benotti PN, Bistrian BR. A clinical application of exercise physiology and nutritional support for the mechanically ventilated patient. *J Parent Enteral Nutr* 1990;**14**:538–42.
116 Rappa D, Lavery R. Psychological dependences on mechanical ventilation resolved by "sigh-breathing" intermittent mandatory ventilation. *Respir Care* 1976;**21**:708–11.
117 Gries ML, Fernsler J. Patient perceptions of the mechanical ventilation experience. *Focus on Critical Care* 1988;**15**:52–9.
118 Kornfield DS, Zimberg S, Malm JE. Psychiatric complications of open-heart surgery. *N Engl J Med* 1965;**273**:287–92.
119 Lazarus LR, Hagens JH. Prevention of psychosis following open-heart surgery. *Am J Psychiatry* 1968;**124**:1190–5.
120 Holland J, Sgroi LSM, Marwit SJ, Solkoff N. The ICU syndrome: fact or fancy? *Psychiatry Med* 1973;**4**:241–9.
121 Kornfield DS, Heller SS, Frank KA, Moskowitz R. Personality and psychological factors in post-cardiotomy delerium. *Arch Gen Psychiatry* 1974;**31**:249–53.
122 Gale J, O'Shanick GJ. Psychiatric aspects of respiratory treatment and pulmonary intensive care. *Adv Psychosom Med* 1985;**14**:93–108.
123 Cronin LR, Carrizosa AA. The computer as a communication device for ventilator and tracheostomy patients in the intensive care unit. *Critical Care Nurse* 1984; Jan–Feb:72–6.
124 Belitz J. Minimising the psychological complications of patients who require mechanical ventilation. *Critical Care Nurse* 1983;May–June:42–6.
125 Helton MC, Gordon SH, Nunnery SL. The correlation between sleep deprivation and the intensive care unit syndrome. *Heart Lung* 1980;**9**:464–8.
126 Cousins MJ, Phillips GD. Sleep, pain and sedation. In: Shoemaker WC, Thomson WC, Holbrook PR, eds *Textbook of critical care*. Philadelphia: Saunders, 1984:797–800.
127 Weissman C, Kemper M, Elwyn DH, Askanazi J, Hyman AI, Kinney JM. The energy expenditure of the mechanically ventilated critically ill patient. *Chest* 1986;**89**:254–9.
128 Bentley S, Murphy F, Dudley H. Perceived noise in surgical wards and an intensive care area: an objective analysis. *Br Med J* 1977;**ii**:1503–6.
129 Redding JS, Hargest TS, Minsky SH. How noisy is intensive care? *Crit Care Med* 1977; **5**:275–6.

4 Weaning from mechanical ventilation

JOHN GOLDSTONE, JOHN MOXHAM

The ability to ventilate the lungs mechanically has led to the widespread application of this technique in the intensive care unit, where the number of patients ventilated and surviving has been steadily increasing since the early 1950s.[1] The indications for ventilatory support are broad (see chapter 2) and include postoperative ventilation, cardiac failure, trauma, and ventilatory support in multiorgan failure in addition to ventilation for respiratory failure.[2] During recovery, the transition from a positive pressure system (on the ventilator) to spontaneous, negative pressure breathing is generally accomplished without difficulty. Drugs are withdrawn, and the patient is allowed to make spontaneous efforts to breathe, either through the ventilator or from a simple breathing circuit. After a trial of unassisted breathing extubation usually follows, with or without supplemental oxygen.

The patient's ability to breathe spontaneously after mechanical ventilation is determined by many factors, including the diagnosis on admission and the length of time spent on the ventilator. The cause of respiratory failure influences outcome and weaning time. In patients with severe COPD, those with exacerbations are remarkably quick to wean compared with patients with underlying infections. In patients receiving short term ventilation 20% of initial trials of spontaneous respiration may not be successful[3] and further ventilation[4] or reintubation will be required.[5] The incidence of weaning failure varies considerably; in a study of patients ventilated after cardiac surgery, where the period of elective ventilation had been a few hours, the overall incidence of initial failure to extubate was as low as 4%.[6]

Although 20% of patients ventilated acutely fail to be weaned initially, their progress and subsequent weaning is usually successful and rapid. Nett and coworkers showed that in such patients over 91% were able to breathe spontaneously after 7 days.[7] In patients in whom weaning was still being attempted at one week the

TABLE 4.1—Physiological measures conventionally associated with weaning failure

Tidal volume	<5 ml/kg[9]
Vital capacity	<10 ml/kg[10]
Minute ventilation (VE)	>10 l/min[11 12]
Maximum voluntary ventilation	<2 × VE[4 13]
Maximum inspiratory pressure	> −20 cm H_2O[4]
Alveolar–arterial oxygen tension difference	>300 mm Hg[14]
Dead space/tidal volume	>0.6[14]

Conversion to SI units: 1 mm Hg = 0.133 kPa; 1 cm H_2O = 0.098 kPa.

problems were complex. This small group, 2% of the total, consisted of patients with pre-existing lung disease as well as those patients surviving after severe multiorgan failure or neuromuscular disease. Patients who receive ventilation for prolonged periods are more likely to require many days for weaning, and may take days or months to achieve spontaneous respiration by day and night.[8]

How then can we decide whether or not a patient is ready to be weaned successfully? This problem was originally studied by investigators measuring respiratory function before and during weaning (table 4.1). Although this approach led to reports of indices which predicted failure, much subsequent work has been contradictory and to date there is no one parameter which can predict successful weaning.

It has been suggested that clinical signs can detect patients who will fail to be weaned, these include rapid shallow breathing[15] and respiratory paradox and alternans.[16] Although such clinical assessment is widely practised, in only about half of the studies is failure to wean associated with increasing tachypnoea.[5 8 14 17 18] Yang and Tobin have quantified rapid shallow breathing in a heterogeneous group of patients admitted to the intensive care unit.[19] Respiratory rate (f) was divided by tidal volume (V_T measured in litres) to give a ratio (f/V_T) which is normally less than 30 (for example 12/0.7 = 17.1). This measure of rapid shallow breathing was then compared with standard tests such as maximum voluntary ventilation (MVV); maximum inspiratory pressure (MIP) and dynamic compliance. The commonly quoted weaning indices (P_{Imax} and minute ventilation, VE) had little specificity for weaning success. The f/V_T ratio was not only highly specific (few patients failed to wean when f/V_T indicated a favourable outcome) but it was also very sensitive (patients who failed had an abnormal f/V_T). When f/V_T exceeded 105, weaning was unlikely. When f/V_T was

TABLE 4.2—A suggested technique for measuring the f/Vt ratio

- Avoid hyperventilation prior to weaning trial
- Remove patient from mechanical support completely
- Use a level of CPAP equivalent to previously required PEEP
- Measure respiratory rate at 5 minutes
- Measure tidal volume at the same FIO_2 (hyperventilation may occur if FIO_2 is transiently decreased during Vt estimation)

less than 80, patients were successfully weaned. These two thresholds can therefore be used in the assessment and quantification of rapid shallow breathing and to predict the outcome of weaning (table 4.2).

Rapid shallow breathing appears to identify patients in the intensive care unit who will fail to wean. It is then important to detect the causes of failure in order to optimise performance and enhance further weaning attempts.

Although weaning is attempted at the earliest opportunity, in patients who have required ventilation for many days it is unlikely that the process will be rapid. Frequent attempts at weaning should be avoided. This was demonstrated by Morganroth and coworkers who studied patients who had been ventilated for many weeks and were difficult to wean.[8] When these patients were able to breathe for only a few hours each day, several more days of assisted ventilation were required (figure 4.1).

Mechanisms of ventilatory failure

The ability to breathe spontaneously depends on three factors: the capacity of the respiratory muscles; the load placed on the respiratory muscle pump; and the central respiratory drive (figure 4. 2). Hypercapnic respiratory failure will ensue when the balance between these factors is disrupted, either by a decrease in capacity (for example, in neuromuscular disease), an increase in load (for example, increased bronchospasm), or depression of central drive (for example, after a drug overdose). When deciding when to withdraw mechanical ventilation, and for how long, and when to reinstitute support, the decision should be made following an assessment of these three components – capacity, load, and drive.

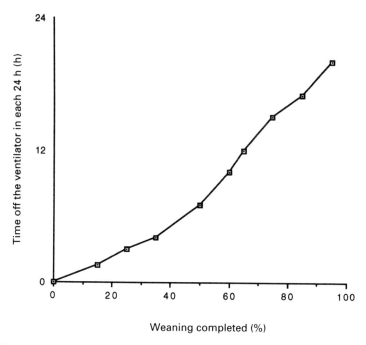

FIG 4.1—In nine patients recovering from critical illness, the total time off the ventilator in each 24 hours is measured against the total duration of weaning and expressed as a percentage. When a patient can only breathe for a few hours, weaning is unlikely to occur quickly, and care must be taken not to withdraw mechanical ventilation too soon. If a patient can breathe for 12 hours unassisted, weaning is almost completed. Taken from Morganroth et al.[8]

Capacity of the respiratory muscles

The capacity of the inspiratory muscles is measured by assessing their ability to generate pressure. Strength can be measured during a static effort against a closed airway and the negative pressure can be recorded at the mouth or in the endotracheal tube (maximum inspiratory pressure, PImax). Most reports of maximum pressure generation in the intensive care unit show a large, up to 75%, reduction in capacity.[41720]

Measuring muscle strength is not straightforward in ventilated patients. Maximum inspiratory pressure is best measured in patients who are alert and cooperative but many patients find it difficult to perform inspiratory manoeuvres which require breath holding, such as a PImax manoeuvre. In order to measure maximum negative

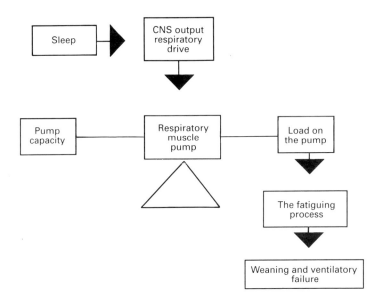

FIG 4.2—Illustration of the central importance of the respiratory muscle pump and the crucial balance between load and capacity. When the ratio of load to capacity is high, the fatiguing process may be initiated, with weaning and ventilatory failure. For successful weaning, adequate respiratory drive must be sustained during sleep as well as when the patient is awake.

pressure generation in the intensive care unit, Marini connected a one-way valve to the endotracheal tube, which allowed expiration but obstructed inspiration.[21] As patients made rapid breathing efforts, functional residual capacity progressively fell and inspiratory effort increased, with maximum inspiratory pressure being achieved by five or six gasps. In a critical review, Multz and coworkers demonstrated that the conventional PImax manoeuvre and the Marini technique produce variable results.[22] The results obtained were often quite different, both between observers and when the same observer measured patients on different days (figure 4.3). When measuring maximum inspiratory pressures it is vital that the patient should achieve maximum drive to the muscles in order to distinguish between weakness of the *peripheral muscles* and inadequate effort. Overventilation and consequent hypocapnia

61

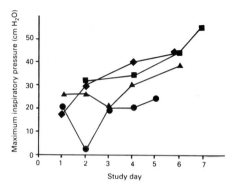

FIG 4.3—Maximum inspiratory pressure measured in four patients on different days by the same observer under the same conditions. Since the patients' respiratory disease was stable, only the highest result can be accurate and the preceding values must be artefactually low. Effort has to be high to achieve maximal results. Taken from Multz et al.[22]

prior to the test may decrease drive and therefore care needs to be taken when testing patients if they are fully ventilated. This problem can be avoided if the patient is able to breathe spontaneously before testing. Effort can be enhanced through verbal encouragement and adequate rest between attempts. Although low pressures may or may not indicate weakness, a large negative pressure (over 45 cm H_2O) indicates that weakness is unlikely to be the main reason for weaning failure. With the Marini technique gasps can be facilitated by using a standard disposable PEEP valve connected to a catheter mount in such a way that the patient can exhale but subsequent inspiratory efforts are occluded. Bedside pressure transducers designed to measure arterial pressure are ideal for measuring airway pressure when filled with air and can be connected via Luer fittings (designed to sample carbon dioxide) to the endotracheal tube. A suitable range of pressures for detecting weakness can be selected

FIG 4.4—Top Set up for measuring maximum inspiratory pressures in an intubated patient: a PEEP valve is attached to the endotracheal tube, allowing expiration but obstructing inspiration. Pressure is measured at the end of the endotracheal tube via a catheter connected to a conventional vascular pressure transducer, and displayed on the bedside monitor. Bottom The trace illustrates progressively greater negative pressures produced by a series of inspiratory gasps. Patients are encouraged to make maximum efforts.

by adjusting the monitor to measure low pressures (for example when measuring central venous pressure). The position of the pressure tracing on the screen needs to be offset as most monitors are not designed to measure negative pressures. Most disposable transducers are differential and therefore one side of the transducer is open to the atmosphere. This can be used to apply a positive pressure to the transducer, and the pressure waveform displayed

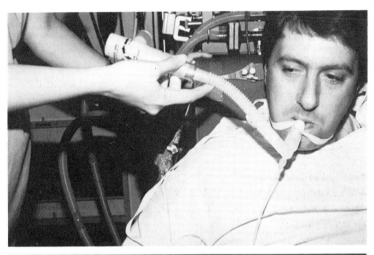

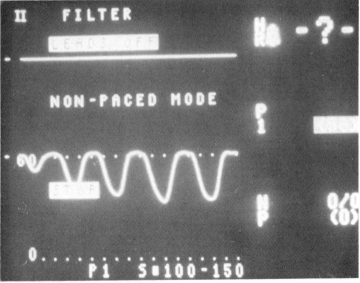

TABLE 4.3—Factors that may impair respiratory muscle contractility in patients in the intensive care unit

---

Hypophosphataemia[27]
Hypomagnesaemia[28]
Hypocalcaemia[29]

Hypoxia
Hypercapnia[30]
Acidosis

Infection[31 32]

Disuse atrophy[33]

Malnutrition[34]

---

can therefore be offset upwards. Negative pressures can then be visualised and estimated (figure 4.4).

Causes of weakness

Patients may be weak prior to admission to the intensive care unit. Systemic disease may affect the respiratory muscles, at the level of the nerves,[23 24] the neuromuscular junction[25] or the muscle itself.[26] This may exacerbate or precipitate respiratory failure. Pulmonary disease may adversely affect the mechanical performance of the respiratory muscles. With airway obstruction there is hyperinflation, muscle shortening, and a reduced capacity to generate inspiratory pressures. When low and flat the diaphragm is less effective at reducing pleural pressure and less able to raise gastric pressure and displace the abdominal contents to achieve a change in volume.

Respiratory muscle strength may diminish after admission to the intensive care unit (table 4.3). Metabolic abnormalities such as hypophosphataemia,[27] hypomagnesaemia,[28] and hypocalcaemia[29] may reduce muscle contractility acutely. The effect of hypoxaemia on muscle function is difficult to assess. Blood flow to muscle increases during hypoxaemia and may offset the decreased carriage of oxygen by blood, thereby maintaining oxygen delivery. In a carefully designed study, Ameredes *et al*[35] showed no change in muscle function during hypoxaemic conditions. Hypercapnia, however, decreases contractility[36] especially if combined with acidosis. Hypoxia and hypercapnia may cause a synergistic decrease in force, as has been found in an animal model.[30]

64

TABLE 4.4—Factors increasing the load on the respiratory muscles in patients in the intensive care unit

---

Bronchoconstriction[39]
Left ventricular failure[40]
Hyperinflation[41]
Intrinsic positive end expiratory pressure
Artificial airways[42]
Ventilator circuits

Muscle performance is reduced by infections. Ventilatory failure occurs as a result of respiratory muscle dysfunction in dogs with septicaemic shock.[31] During an upper respiratory tract infection muscle performance measured in terms of maximum inspiratory and expiratory mouth pressures is reduced by 30%.[32] Muscle atrophy occurs with disuse,[37] and this may be accelerated by sepsis. Anzueto et al[33] ventilated primates artificially and found after 11 days that diaphragm strength, measured during phrenic nerve stimulation, was reduced by 46%. Malnutrition occurs in many patients before admission to the intensive care unit, and may continue during the intercurrent illness. Respiratory muscle strength is reduced in undernourished patients[38] and the mass of the diaphragm is decreased in patients who are wasted.[34]

Load

During mechanical ventilation the work of breathing is performed by the ventilator and is dissipated during gas compression, overcoming airflow resistance, and inflating the chest against the elastic recoil of the lung and chest wall. Some energy is expended during the breathing cycle that does not contribute to gas flow but results in the deformation of the chest wall. Although this may be substantial, the load applied to the respiratory muscles is largely related to the elastic and resistive elements during gas flow. In the intensive care unit the ventilatory load is often much higher than normal (table 4.4).

Causes of increased load

Load can be increased substantially by airway obstruction. During asthma induced by histamine challenge a fall in FEV_1 of 40% is associated with a threefold increase in load which requires an eightfold increase in pressure generation per tidal breath.[43] In patients ventilated for left ventricular failure, Rossi et al[44] measured

65

compliance and airway resistance, and showed a substantial increase in the load imposed on the respiratory muscles. Resting oxygen consumption is increased in chronic airflow limitation, reflecting the increased work of breathing,[45] and in patients in left ventricular failure being weaned from ventilators the oxygen cost of breathing is four times greater than normal.[39] Left ventricular function is impaired in many patients admitted to the intensive care unit, and pulmonary oedema increases the load substantially. This may occur during the transition to negative pressure breathing, as positive pressure ventilation may act to assist the left ventricle via transmitted pressure from the ventilator to the chambers of the heart.[40,46]

During weaning, patients breathe through airways and ventilators, and this increases the load substantially.[47] The work required to breathe through an artificial airway is large,[48] greater than the work of breathing through the upper airway alone,[49] and it may double the load applied to the system.[50] The work needed to breathe through a tracheostomy may equal the work of breathing through the longer oral endotracheal tubes,[42] and may itself prevent spontaneous respiration.[51] Increased work is performed when patients are breathing through many circuits, especially when they are required to open valves to achieve inspiration.[52]

In many ventilated patients, especially those with airflow limitation, the time for expiration may not allow complete exhalation to functional residual capacity. Subsequent tidal breaths increase end expiratory volume and pressure; this is termed intrinsic or auto PEEP. During a spontaneous breath the increased elastic recoil pressure of the lungs and chest wall must be overcome, and in patients who are weak this may be as much as half of their maximum inspiratory pressure generating capacity, thus intrinsic PEEP imposes a large additional load on the respiratory muscles.[53] Fiastro et al[54] measured the work of breathing during weaning from mechanical ventilation and found that patients able to breathe spontaneously had less work to perform than those who failed. In the "failed" group, spontaneous respiration was achieved only when respiratory work was reduced to that observed in the successful group.

Measurement of the load applied to the respiratory system
In mechanically ventilated, relaxed patients the ventilator provides all the motive power to inflate the lung and move the chest wall.

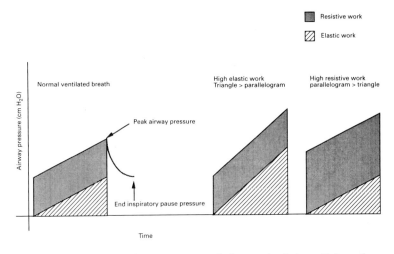

FIG 4.5—Stylised traces of airway pressure during mechanical ventilation where the patient is completely relaxed. If the ventilator is a flow generator, the area under the pressure–time diagrams equals the work performed during the breath. Compare the normal breath with the large triangular area seen when the elastic work is high (stiff lungs, for example in ARDS) and with the large parallelogram seen when the resistive work is high (for example in asthma).

Work is measured from the product of pressure and volume and is commonly assessed in the laboratory by integrating a pressure–volume plot during lung inflation.

Work can be measured at the bedside by assessing the area under the graph of airway pressure against time. Pressure can be measured by air-filled transducers as described earlier, and the positive pressure waveforms require no adjustment to be displayed on bedside monitors. As most intensive care unit ventilators are constant flow generators (see chapter 1), the time axis equates linearly to volume delivered by the ventilator. The area under such a graph is therefore a pressure–volume curve and represents the work performed by the ventilator. Marini and coworkers[55] assessed the work measured from such waveforms at the bedside and found close agreement between this and conventional measurements under different inspiratory flow rates (figure 4.5).

Respiratory mechanics can be assessed from these diagrams and dynamic compliance calculated (inspiratory volume/peak airway pressure − PEEP). In addition the shape of the airway pressure–time diagrams is changed when resistive or elastic loads predominate.[57]

Such diagrams therefore provide a graphic method of monitoring the response to bronchodilator therapy. Several modern ventilators can provide a display of airway pressure which can be monitored at the bedside.

Central drive

Force generation of the respiratory muscles is related to output from the central nervous system in terms of the number of contractile units activated and the motor neurone firing frequency. In health and at rest, low levels of central drive and concomitant low motor neurone firing frequencies are sufficient to effect an adequate tidal volume; in contrast, patients with chronic respiratory failure have higher respiratory drives.[41][58]

Failure to breathe spontaneously during weaning has been correlated with an increased central drive that cannot be sustained.[59] Although occasional studies have shown that respiratory drive is reduced and may respond to central stimulants,[60] this has not been observed in most investigations. In a recent investigation in patients with COPD[61] doxapram administration did not alter ventilatory drive or minute ventilation, but was responsible for a rise in FRC which would, if anything, worsen ventilatory function.

It is difficult to measure drive at the bedside, and the conventional method (the pressure generated after 100 ms of an occluded inspiration, P0.1) is an indirect index which is frequently difficult to interpret.

The load: capacity balance: respiratory muscle fatigue

When the load applied to the respiratory muscles exceeds their capacity to generate pressure the likely outcome is the development of hypercapnic ventilatory failure, leading to acidosis, coma, and death. The hypothesis is that in these circumstances the respiratory muscles cannot sustain the required pressures without fatigue (see figure 4.2).

Evidence supporting this hypothesis has largely come from studies in normal subjects breathing through inspiratory resistances. It has been shown that ventilation cannot be sustained when the pressure generated per breath exceeds 40% of maximum pressure.[62] The ability to maintain ventilation is also related to the duration of contraction of the inspiratory muscles during each breath. Bellemare and Grassino[63] performed repeated trials of inspiratory resistive loading measuring the time of inspiration (Ti) as a fraction of the respiratory cycle (Ttot). They defined the relationship between the strength of the diaphragm (Pdi max) and the duration and fraction of maximum pressure generated during each breath:

$$\text{Tension–time index} = \frac{\text{Pdi}}{\text{Pdi max}} \times \frac{\text{Ti}}{\text{Ttot}}$$

This tension–time index is about 0·05 during resting ventilation. When it exceeds 0·15, through an increase either in the duration of inspiration or inspiratory pressure (induced experimentally by breathing through a resistance), ventilation cannot be sustained. Few studies have measured the tension–time index in the intensive care unit during weaning. Pourriat and coworkers[18] however, showed that patients who could not be weaned required a greater fraction of their maximum inspiratory pressure during each breath.

The relation between load, capacity, and fatigue in patients in the intensive care unit has been studied in terms of a modified tension–time index, the inspiratory effort quotient.[64] The mean pressure developed during inspiration is determined by tidal volume (VT) and dynamic compliance (Cdyn), and depends also on the shape of the inspiratory pressure curve (K):

$$\text{Inspiratory effort quotient} = \frac{\text{KVt/Cdyn}}{\text{Pimax}} \times \frac{\text{Ti}}{\text{Ttot}}$$

It has been demonstrated that the inspiratory effort quotient is low in patients who wean from mechanical ventilation.[65] When the quotient exceeds 0.23, weaning is unlikely[66] (figure 4.6). This suggests that successful weaning is related to the balance between the strength of the respiratory muscles and the load applied to them rather than the absolute value of either measure. This may explain the variable predictive power in studies where aspects of strength or load are measured alone.

Given that excessive load in relation to capacity may lead to fatigue, a measurement of fatigue could be used to monitor patients being weaned from mechanical ventilation. This would enable patients to be reventilated at an appropriate moment, before the development of hypercapnia. With established fatigue, maximum inspiratory pressures are reduced but measuring them in patients

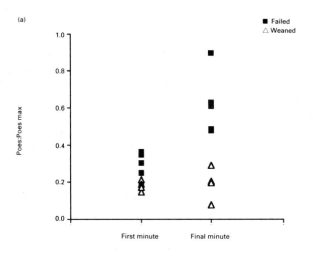

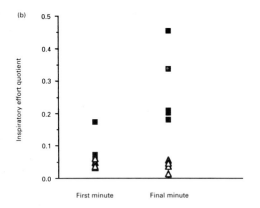

FIG 4.6—The balance between load and strength numerically expressed in (a) as Poes:Poes max ratio and in (b) as the inspiratory effort quotient measured at the first minute off the ventilator and at the end of trials of weaning in nine patients. Both Poes:Poes max and the IEQ were high in the five patients who failed to wean, indicating that the load applied to the respiratory muscles exceeded their capacity. Taken from Goldstone et al.[65]

in the intensive care unit has hitherto been difficult and the results are variable.

During muscular activity of an intensity sufficient to lead to fatigue the speed of contraction and relaxation of muscle slows.[67] During a brief inspiratory sniff the rate of relaxation of the respiratory muscles can be measured in terms of the maximum relaxation rate of oesophageal pressure.[68] In normal subjects, during fatigue induced by loaded ventilation the maximum relaxation rate slows, and recovers rapidly with rest. Patients in the intensive care unit are usually intubated, with their upper airway bypassed, and unable to perform a sniff. A device that enables intubated patients to perform a sniff-like manoeuvre has been used recently to study patients in the intensive care unit.[65] In those who could not be weaned the maximum relaxation rate slowed progressively and recovered after reventilation, suggesting that fatigue of the respiratory muscles was occurring during the attempt at weaning. Patients weaned successfully showed no slowing of the maximum relaxation rate of the respiratory muscles. In the future, when patients being weaned from mechanical ventilation are being assessed and monitored, the maximum relaxation rate could perhaps be used as a reflection of the relation between the capacity of the respiratory muscles and the load that is applied to them. Slowing of the maximum relaxation rate could provide an early indication that weaning will fail.

A strategy for weaning

It is important that patients who have failed to wean are identified at an early stage, because repetitive failure is a distressing and unproductive exercise. The end point of a trial of weaning should not be the development of hypercapnic acidosis. When the causative factors that precipitated the need for ventilation are reversed, the patient may be ready for weaning. Weaning is more likely to succeed in an alert, rested, cooperative patient. Sedation, confusion, and tiredness will make weaning less likely. In alert patients central respiratory drive is likely to be optimal; respiratory stimulants are of limited value and potentially harmful.

Optimising respiratory muscle capacity

In general, patients in the intensive care unit are weak, and small changes made to improve their strength or to reduce the

71

load applied to the weakened respiratory muscles will be beneficial.

Correction of hypophosphataemia has been shown to increase strength and to facilitate weaning.[69] Electrolyte abnormalities should also be corrected. Although there is no direct evidence that hypercapnia and hypoxaemia affect weaning, respiratory muscle function is likely to be reduced if the patient is acidotic, and tissue acidosis may be intensified by hypoxaemia. Nutritional support should be provided in the intensive care unit. Patients are often undernourished before admission to hospital, and the deficit may be large. Uptake of nutritional substrates may be impaired during episodes of critical illness, and intravenous feeding may be difficult in patients with complex fluid balance problems. Patients can seldom be weaned during septic episodes, and weaning failure is more likely in patients with a positive blood culture.[5] Respiratory muscle function may be diminished substantially by endotoxaemia. Although drugs, particularly aminophylline, have been reported to enhance respiratory muscle performance,[70] the balance of evidence suggests this is not the case.[71]

Minimising the ventilatory load

During weaning the load applied to the muscles may alter acutely, precipitating respiratory failure and the need for reventilation.[54] Patients may have fluid overload or hypoalbuminaemia, leading to pulmonary oedema at relatively low filling pressures. The mechanical enhancement of left ventricular performance by ventilation and the changes during weaning require consideration.

Airway obstruction increases the respiratory load and decreases respiratory muscle performance, and should be treated aggressively. Patients may be stable when assessed during mechanical ventilation yet develop wheeze during spontaneous breathing, and should therefore be assessed during the weaning trial. Hyperinflation is likely in patients with airway obstruction, and may be exacerbated by mechanical ventilation, which may increase intrinsic positive end expiratory pressure. Over-distension during mechanical ventilation can be monitored simply by displaying airway pressure during intermittent positive pressure ventilation on the bedside monitor, and watching for the characteristic waveform seen in such patients.[57] Intrinsic positive end expiratory pressure can be measured by occluding the expiratory limb of the ventilator during a prolonged expiratory pause, and measuring the airway pressure transmitted to the pressure gauge of the ventilator.[72] Patients susceptible to hyperinflation may breathe more effectively when removed from the ventilator altogether rather than weaning with intermittent mandatory ventilation.[73]

Breathing apparatus may impose a substantial respiratory load on patients. Resistance to flow increases with decreased tube diameter, and with a high minute ventilation may impose an unsustainable tension–time index of more than $0 \cdot 15$.[48] This load can be overcome by using inspiratory pressure support.

The benefit of PEEP is difficult to assess in the hyperinflated patient[74] and when used should not exceed the measured auto-PEEP.[75] PEEP is of value in patients who have muscle weakness or obesity, or postoperative basal collapse. In such patients it increases functional residual capacity, prevents airway closure and atelectasis, increases compliance, and reduces ventilatory work. In these circumstances weaning is usually facilitated by adding CPAP.

Much attention has been focused on the method of weaning patients from the ventilator, and opinion is divided. One method is to allow the patient to breathe spontaneously via a T-piece circuit for gradually lengthening periods with full ventilation between them. An alternative approach is to provide partial respiratory support through the ventilator and to allow the patient to breathe spontaneously between mechanical breaths (SIMV see chapter 2 for the different techniques of ventilation and support). IPS is a pressure limited mode of ventilation which is triggered by inspiratory effort and maintains a preset positive airway pressure until the flow rate decreases and this terminates inspiration. Currently there is no evidence to suggest that any method is markedly superior (see below).[76]

General measures

Weaning, especially in patients who have been ventilated for many days or weeks, may be a great burden both physically and mentally. Sleep may be lost and disrupted and morale low, especially if the patient feels "stuck" on the ventilator. Although daytime respiratory drive should not be depressed, the establishment of regular sleeping patterns may require short acting sedative drugs.

The endpoint of a weaning trial is difficult to assess in some patients, as there are no current guidelines as to when reventilation is mandatory, though the development of hypercapnia and acidosis indicates that reventilation is necessary. In studies of high intensity workloads in skeletal muscle, biopsy material has shown necrosis[77] and such changes probably occur in respiratory muscles if they are sufficiently stressed. Damage to the respiratory muscles, especially in patients who have severe weakness, will impede successful weaning. In addition, breathing to the point of exhaustion demoralises the patient, erodes previous progress, and is therefore counterproductive.

Monitoring during weaning

Although investigators have sought to identify parameters which predict weaning failure, few have addressed the question of how long a patient should be weaned for and when they should be reventilated. While tachypnoea is an early sign of eventual failure,[15] patients with tachypnoea can often breathe for substantial periods unassisted. Gandia and Blanco[66] have assessed rapid shallow breathing by measuring f/VT at 15, 60 and 120 minutes and found that whereas f/VT distinguished those who weaned successfully from those who did not, no changes in f/VT occurred over the 2 hour period, suggesting that as a monitor of the *end point* of weaning f/VT may not be helpful.

Those patients with critical left ventricular function are a particular problem. This should be suspected in patients who repeatedly fail to wean. Poor cardiac output may be detected during spontaneous breathing by echocardiography or cardiac output measurements despite a steady state during assisted ventilation.

Modes of weaning and new ventilatory techniques

Intermittent mandatory ventilation was used to wean adults[78] after its successful application in neonates to enable patients to breathe spontaneously while receiving volume controlled ventilation. The technique was subsequently modified so that machine inflation coincided with SIMV, thereby avoiding high airway pressures.

Ventilators can be regarded as machines which off load respiratory muscles. However the extent of this off loading is difficult to judge. In non-paralysed patients the respiratory muscles contract even during controlled machine breathing at a level that can be similar to that found in patients breathing spontaneously.[79] This is clinically apparent when spontaneous breathing is not synchronous, when there is a large time delay between muscle contraction and ventilator cycling, or in patients where high resistance prevents the ventilator from detecting each breath. It also occurs when the

74

ventilator cannot quickly deliver a high enough flow rate or when the preset flow rate is insufficient.

Although it was first envisaged that SIMV would decrease weaning time this is probably not the case. Tomlinson and coworkers have demonstrated that in patients weaned after short periods of mechanical ventilation there is no difference between SIMV and simple T-piece weaning.[76]

IPS is a form of pressure controlled ventilation which is entirely dependent on the patient's breathing effort. As inspiration is sensed, a high inspiratory flow rate occurs until the pressure generated in the airway achieves the target pressure. With rapidly opening valves ventilation is achieved with little delay and IPS is well tolerated. Although IPS reduces the electrical evidence of diaphragmatic fatigue,[80] this can also be achieved with volume controlled ventilation,[16] albeit with greater difficulty; a prospective, controlled trial of IPS during weaning has yet to be reported.

Low levels (5 cm H_2O) of IPS can offset the work performed when breathing through tubes and connectors.[81] Minimal pressure support can be calculated from the peak inspiratory flow rate and overall respiratory resistance (PIFR × R).[82] In order to reduce the work imposed by demand valves, Flow-By is a mode of ventilation which allows patients to breathe through circuits with minimal effort; it is comparable to 5 cm H_2O IPS in a demand valve CPAP system.[83]

IPS is a patient controlled mode of ventilation and it is therefore poorly suited to patients with a variable respiratory drive or changing lung mechanics. In both circumstances reductions in tidal volume will occur. Volume assured pressure support ventilation (VAPSV) combines an inspiratory flow pattern similar to IPS, via a low impedance, high flow system, with a conventional constant flow, high impedance gas source operating in series.[84] The high flow gas supply reduces the "flow starvation" seen in volume cycled ventilation and inspiratory work can be halved compared with volume controlled ventilation. In addition, as respiratory effort is reduced, the system is able to rely on the constant flow gas supply to ensure a preset tidal volume.

Further progress in matching ventilator performance to the needs of patients will come from refining the ability of the ventilator to sense the beginning of inspiration. Ideally, inspiration should occur at the beginning of muscular contraction, reducing inspiratory work to a minimum. In many patients who trigger ventilation, significant work occurs, especially if the triggering pressure has to be transmitted along the breathing circuit to the ventilator. This problem is worsened by poor lung mechanics, especially if airways resistance is high. Takahashi and coworkers[85] have investigated a lung model in which the trigger is moved from the ventilator to the pleural space, with the ventilator in pressure support mode (pleural pressure support ventilation, PPSV). This considerably reduces the work of breathing and the time taken for the ventilator to trigger is substantially less, and is largely unaffected by alterations to lung resistance or dynamic compliance.

A small number of patients who are difficult to wean can be successfully managed by non-invasive nasal or facemask ventilation NIPPV (see Chapter 5). This technique enables selected patients to be extubated after a short adaptive period and has been successfully applied to long stay patients in the intensive care unit.[86] It allows many patients to be nursed less intensively, facilitates eating and drinking and may avoid the need for tracheostomy.

1 Snider GL. Historical perspective on mechanical ventilation: from simple life support system to ethical dilemma. *Am Rev Resp Dis* 1989;**140**:S2–S7.

2 Braun NMT. Intermittent mechanical ventilation. *Clin Chest Med* 1988;**9**:153–62.

3 Hilberman M, Kamm B, Lamy M, Dietrich HP, Martz K, Osborn JJ. An analysis of potential physiological predictors of respiratory adequacy following cardiac surgery. *J Thorac Cardiovasc Surg* 1976;**71**:711–20.

4 Sahn SA, Lakshminarayan S. Bedside criteria for discontinuation of mechanical ventilation. *Chest* 1973;**63**:1002–5.

5 Tahvanainen J, Salmenpera M, Nikki P. Extubation criteria after weaning from intermittent mandatory ventilation and continuous positive airway pressure. *Crit Care Med* 1983;**11**: 702–7.

6 Demling RH, Read T, Lind LJ, Flanagan HL. Incidence and morbidity of extubation failure in surgical intensive care patients. *Crit Care Med* 1988;**16**:573–7.

7 Nett LM, Morganroth M, Petty TL. Weaning from mechanical ventilation: a perspective and review of techniques. In: Bone RC ed. *Critical care: a comprehensive approach.* Park Ridge, IL: American College of Chest Physicians, 1984:171–88.

8 Morganroth ML, Morganroth JL, Nett LM. Criteria for weaning from prolonged mechanical ventilation. *Arch Int Med* 1984;**144**:1012–6.

9 Radford EP, Ferris BG, Kriete BC. Clinical use of a nomogram to estimate proper ventilation during artificial ventilation. *N Eng J Med* 1954;**251**:877–84.

10 Bendixen HH, Egbert LD, Hedley-White J. Management of patients undergoing prolonged artificial ventilation. In: *Respiratory care.* St Louis: CV Mosby and Co, 1965:149–50.

11 Aldrich TK, Karpel JP. Inspiratory muscle resistive training in respiratory failure. *Am Rev Respir Dis* 1985;**131**:461–2.

12 Aldrich TK, Uhrlass RM. Weaning from mechanical ventilation: Successful use of modified inspiratory resistive training in muscular dystrophy. *Crit Care Med* 1987;**15**:247–9.

13 Stetson JB. *Prolonged tracheal intubation.* Boston: Little Brown and Co, 1970:767–79.

14 Pontoppidan H, Laver MB, Geffin B. Acute respiratory failure in the surgical patient. In: Welch CE, ed. *Advances in surgery.* Vol 4. Chicago: Year Book Medical Publishers, 1970: 163–254.

15 Tobin MJ, Peres W, Guenther SM, et al. The pattern of breathing during successful and unsuccessful trials of weaning from mechanical ventilation. *Am Rev Respir Dis* 1986;**134**: 1111–8.

16 Cohen CA, Zagelbaum G, Gross D, Roussos C, Macklem PT. Clinical manifestations of inspiratory muscle fatigue. *Am J Med* 1982;73:308–16.
17 Kacmarek RM, Cycyk-Chapman MC, Young-Palazzo PJ, Romagnoli DM. Determination of maximum inspiratory pressure: A clinical study and literature review. *Resp Care* 1989; 34:868–78.
18 Pourriat JL, Lamberto C, Hoang PH, Fournier JL, Vasseur B. Diaphragmatic fatigue and breathing pattern during weaning from mechanical ventilation in COPD patients. *Chest* 1986;90:703–7.
19 Yang KL, Tobin MJ. A prospective study of indexes predicting the outcome of trials of weaning from mechanical ventilation. *N Eng J Med* 1991;324:1445–50.
20 Krieger BP, Ershowsky PF, Becker DA, Gazeroglu HB. Evaluation of conventional criteria for predicting successful weaning from mechanical ventilatory support in elderly patients. *Crit Care Med* 1989;17:858–61.
21 Marini JJ, Smith TC, Lamb V. Estimation of inspiratory muscle strength in mechanically ventilated patients: measurement of maximum inspiratory pressure. *J Crit Care* 1988;1: 32–8.
22 Multz AS, Aldrich TK, Prezant DJ, Karpel JP, Hendler JM. Maximal inspiratory pressure is not a reliable test of inspiratory muscle strength in mechanically ventilated patients. *Am Rev Respir Dis* 1990;142:529–32.
23 Cooper CB, Trend PSJ, Wiles CM. Severe diaphragm weakness in multiple sclerosis. *Thorax* 1985;40:633–4.
24 Al-Shaikh B, Kinnear W, Higgenbottam TW, Smith HS, Sneerson JM, Wilkinson I. Motor neurone disease presenting as respiratory failure. *Br Med J* 1986;292:1325–6.
25 Mier A, Brophy C, Green M. Respiratory muscle function in myasthenia gravis. *Am Rev Respir Dis* 1988;138:867–73.
26 Braun NMT, Arora NS, Rochester DF. Respiratory muscle and pulmonary function in polymyositis and other proximal myopathies. *Thorax* 1983;38:616–23.
27 Newman JH, Neff TA, Ziporin P. Acute respiratory failure associated with hypophosphatemia. *N Engl J Med* 1977;296:1101–3.
28 Dhingra S, Solven F, Wilson A, McCathy D. Hypomagnesemia and respiratory muscle power. *Am Rev Respir Dis* 1984;129:497–8.
29 Aubier M, Viires N, Piquet J, et al. Effects of hypocalcaemia on diaphragmatic strength generation. *J Appl Physiol* 1985;58:2054–61.
30 Esau SA, Hypoxic, hypercapnic acidosis decreases tension and increases fatigue in hamster diaphragm muscle in vitro. *Am Rev Resp Dis* 1989;139:1410–7.
31 Hussain SNA, Simkus G, Roussos C. Respiratory muscle failure: a cause of ventilatory failure in septic shock. *J Appl Physiol* 1985;58:2033–40.
32 Mier-Jedrzejowicz A, Brophy C, Green M. Respiratory muscle weakness during upper respiratory tract infections. *Am Rev Respir Dis* 1988;138:5–7.
33 Anzueto A, Tobin MJ, Moore G. Effect of prolonged mechanical ventilation on diaphragmatic function: A preliminary study of a baboon model. *Am Rev Respir Dis* 1987; 135:A201.
34 Arora NS, Rochester DF. Effect of body weight and muscularity on human diaphragm muscle mass, thickness and area. *J Appl Physiol* 1982;52:64–70.
35 Ameredes BT, Clanton TL. Hyperoxia and moderate hypoxia fail to affect inspiratory muscle fatigue in humans. *J Appl Physiol* 1989;66:894–900.
36 Juan G, Calverley P. Talamo C, Schnader J, Roussos C. Effect of carbon dioxide on diaphragmatic function in human beings. *N Engl J Med* 1984;310:874–9.
37 Musacchia XJ, Deavers DR, Meininger GA, Davis TP. A model for hypokinesia: effects on muscle atrophy in the rat. *J Appl Physiol* 1980;48:479–86.
38 Arora NS, Rochester DF. Respiratory muscle strength and maximum voluntary ventilation in undernourished patients. *Am Rev Respir Dis* 1982;126:5–8.
39 Field S, Kelly SM, Macklem PT. The oxygen cost of breathing in patients with cardiorespiratory disease. *Am Rev Respir Dis* 1982;126:9–13.
40 Beach T, Millen G, Grenvik A. Haemodynamic response to discontinuance of mechanical ventilation. *Crit Care Med* 1973;1:85–90.
41 Gribben HR, Gardiner IT, Heinz CJ, Gibson TJ, Pride NB. The role of impaired inspiratory muscle function in limiting ventilatory response to CO_2 in chronic airflow limitation. *Clin Sci* 1983;64:487–95.
42 Plost J, Campbell JC. The non-elastic work of breathing through endotracheal tubes of various sizes. *Am Rev Respir Dis* 1984;129:A106.

43 Martin JG, Shore SA, Engel LA. Mechanical load and inspiratory muscle action during asthma. *Am Rev Respir Dis* 1983;**128**:455–60.
44 Rossi A, Poggi R, Manzin E, Broseghini C, Brandolese R. Early changes in respiratory mechanics in acute respiratory failure. In: Grassino A, Fracchia C, Rampulla C, Zocchi L, eds. *Respiratory muscles in COPD*. London: Springer Verlag, 1988:149–60.
45 Lanigan C, Moxham J, Ponte J. Effect of chronic airflow limitation on resting oxygen consumption. *Thorax* 1990;**45**:388–90.
46 Robotham JL, Cherry D, Mitzner W, Rabson JL, Lixfield W, Bromberger-Barnea B. A re-evaluation of the hemodynamic consequences of intermittent positive pressure ventilation. *Crit Care Med* 1983;**11**:783–93.
47 Marini JJ. The role of the inspiratory circuit in the work of breathing during mechanical ventilation. *Resp Care* 1987;**32**:419–30.
48 Shapiro M, Wilson RK, Casar G, Bloom K, Teague RB. Work of breathing through different sized endotracheal tubes. *Crit Care Med* 1986;**14**:1028–31.
49 Habib MP. Physiological implications of artificial airways. *Chest* 1989;**96**:181–4.
50 Wright PE, Marini JJ, Bernard GR. In vitro versus in vivo comparison of endotracheal tube airflow resistance. *Am Rev Respir Dis* 1989;**140**:10–6.
51 Criner G, Make B, Celli B. Respiratory muscle dysfunction secondary to chronic tracheostomy tube placement. *Chest* 1987;**91**:139–41.
52 Gibney RTN, Wilson RS, Pontoppidan H. Comparison of work of breathing on high gas flow and demand valve continuous positive airway pressure systems. *Chest* 1982;**82**:692.
53 Kimball WR, Leith DE, Robins AG. Dynamic hyperinflation and ventilator dependence in chronic obstructive pulmonary disease. *Am Rev Respir Dis* 1982;**126**:991–5.
54 Fiastro JF, Habib MP, Shon BY, Cambell SC. Comparison of standard weaning parameters and the mechanical work of breathing in mechanically ventilated patients. *Chest* 1988;**94**:232–8.
55 Marini JJ, Rodriguez RM, Lamb V. Bedside estimation of the inspiratory work of breathing during mechanical ventilation. *Chest* 1986;**89**:56–63.
56 Hubermayr RD, Gay PC, Tayyab M. Respiratory system mechanics in ventilated patients: techniques and indications. *Mayo Clinics Proc* 1987;**62**:358–68.
57 Milic-Emili J, Ploysongsang Y. Respiratory mechanics in the adult respiratory distress syndrome. *Crit Care Clin* 1986;**2**:573–84.
58 Murciano D, Aubier M, Bussi S, Derenne JP, Pariente R, Milic-Emili J. Comparison of eosophageal, tracheal and occlusion pressure in patients with chronic obstructive pulmonary disease during acute respiratory failure. *Am Rev Respir Dis* 1982;**126**:837–41.
59 Herrera M, Blasco J, Venegas J, Barba R, Dublas A, Marquez E. Mouth occlusion pressure (P0.1) in acute respiratory failure. *Inten Care Med* 1985;**11**:134–9.
60 Hoake RE, Saxon LA, Bander SJ, Hoake RJ. Depressed central respiratory drive causing weaning failure. *Chest* 1989;**95**:695–7.
61 Pourriat JL, Baud M, Lamberto C, Fosse JP, Cupa M. Effects of doxapram on hypercapnic response during weaning from mechanical ventilation in COPD patients. *Chest* 1992;**101**:1639–43.
62 Roussos CS, Macklem PT. Diaphragmatic fatigue in man. *J Appl Physiol* 1977;**43**:189–97.
63 Bellemare F, Grassino A. Effect of pressure and timing of contraction on human diaphragm fatigue. *J Appl Physiol* 1982;**53**:1190–5.
64 Milic-Emili J. Is weaning an art or a science? *Am Rev Respir Dis* 1986;**134**:1107–8.
65 Goldstone JC, Green M, Moxham J. Maximum relaxation rate of the diaphragm during weaning from mechanical ventilation. *Thorax* 1994;**49**:54–60.
66 Gandia F, Blanco J. Evaluation of indexes predicting the outcome of ventilator weaning and value of adding supplemental inspiratory load. *Inten Care Med* 1992;**18**:327–33.
67 Esau SA, Bellemare F, Grassino A, Permutt S, Roussos C, Pardy RL. Changes in relaxation rate with diaphragmatic fatigue in humans. *J Appl Physiol* 1983;**54**:1353–60.
68 Koulouris N, Vianna LG, Mulvey DH, Green M, Moxham J. Maximum relaxation rates of esophageal, nose and mouth pressures during a sniff reflect inspiratory muscle fatigue. *Am Rev Respir Dis* 1989;**139**:1213–7.
69 Agusti AGN, Torres A, Estopa R, Agusti-Vidal A. Hypophosphatemia as a cause of failed weaning: The importance of metabolic factors. *Crit Care Med* 1984;**12**:142–3.
70 Aubier M. Pharmacotherapy of respiratory muscles. *Clin Chest Med* 1988;**9**:311–24.
71 Moxham J. Aminophylline and the respiratory muscles; an alternative view. *Clin Chest Med* 1988;**9**:325–36.

72 Pepe PE, Marini JJ. Occult positive end-expiratory pressure in mechanically ventilated patients with airflow obstruction. *Am Rev Respir Dis* 1982;**126**:166–70.
73 Williams MH. IMV and weaning. *Chest* 1980;**78**:804.
74 Marini JJ. Should PEEP be used in airflow limitation? *Am Rev Respir Dis* 1989;**140**:1–3.
75 Tobin MJ, Lodato RF. Peep, Auto-Peep, and waterfalls. *Chest* 1989;**96**:449–51.
76 Tomlinson JR, Scott Miller K, Lorch DG, Smith L, Reines HD, Sahn SA. A prospective comparison of IMV and T-piece weaning from mechanical ventilation. *Chest* 1989;**96**: 348–52.
77 Vihko V, Salminen A, Rantamaki J. Exhaustive exercise, endurance training and acid hydrolase activity in skeletal muscle. *J Appl Physiol* 1979;**47**:43–50.
78 Downs JB, Klein EF, Desautels D, Modell JH, Kirby RR. Intermittent mandatory ventilation: a new approach to weaning patients from mechanical ventilation. *Chest* 1973;**64**:331–5.
79 Flick GR, Bellamy PE, Simmons DH. Diaphragmatic contraction during assisted mechanical ventilation. *Chest* 1989;**96**:130–5.
80 Brochard L, Harf A, Lorino H, Lemaire F. Inspiratory pressure support prevents diaphragmatic fatigue during weaning from mechanical ventilation. *Am Rev Respir Dis* 1989;**139**:513–21.
81 Sassoon CSH, Light RW, Lodia R, Sieck GC, Mahutte CK. Pressure-time product during continuous positive airway pressure, pressure support ventilation and t-piece during weaning from mechanical ventilation. *Am Rev Respir Dis* 1991;**143**:469–75.
82 Nathan SD, Ishaaya AM, Koerner SK, Belman MJ. Prediction of minimal pressure support during weaning from mechanical ventilation. *Chest* 1993;**103**:1215–9.
83 Sassoon CSH, Lodia R, Rheeman CH, Kuie JH, Light RW, Mahutte CK. Inspiratory muscle work of breathing during flow by, demand flow and continuous flow systems in patients with chronic obstructive pulmonary disease. *Am Rev Respir Dis* 1992;**145**: 1219–22.
84 Amato MBP, Barbas CSV, Bonassa J, Saldiva PHN, Zin WA, de Carvalho CRR. Volume-assured pressure support ventilation (VAPSV); a new approach for reducing muscle workload during acute respiratory failure. *Chest* 1992;**102**:1225–34.
85 Takahashi T, Takezawa J, Kimura T, Nishiwaki K, Shimada Y. Comparison of inspiratory work of breathing in t-piece breathing, PSV and pleural pressure support ventilation (PPSV). *Chest* 1991;**100**:1030–4.
86 Udwadia ZF, Santis GK, Steven MH, Simonds AK. Nasal ventilation to facilitate weaning in patients with chronic respiratory insufficiency. *Thorax* 1992;**47**:715–8.

5 Non-invasive ventilation

M W ELLIOTT, A K SIMONDS, JOHN MOXHAM

In the past, patients requiring long term domiciliary ventilation have used negative pressure devices or positive pressure devices associated with a mouth piece or tracheostomy. This has been effective, but expertise has been confined to a few specialist centres and relatively few patients have been treated. With the recognition that positive pressure ventilation could be delivered through a nasal mask, and the availability of relatively cheap ventilators suitable for home use, the frequency of domiciliary support has increased greatly. With improvements in equipment and greater understanding of the technique, the indications for domiciliary nasal positive pressure ventilation (NPPV) have widened and now include some patients with hypercapnic respiratory failure associated with intrinsic lung disease. Additionally NPPV has been used in hospital to treat patients with acute on chronic respiratory failure reducing the need for intubation and admission to the intensive care unit. If patients have been intubated and it is difficult to wean them from mechanical ventilation, NPPV may be used to facilitate the resumption of spontaneous breathing.

NPPV is now the mode of choice for non-invasive ventilation, however, negative pressure devices may be preferred by some patients,[1] particularly those who find a mask and head gear claustrophobic or are troubled by painful gastric distension with NPPV. Negative pressure devices are relatively inefficient, particularly when the impedance to inflation is high, and they predispose to upper airway obstruction.[2] The tank ventilator is the most effective negative pressure device, but there may be problems in achieving an adequate seal around the neck and though ports allow access to the patient, routine nursing care is difficult. Simpler less expensive devices, such as cuirass and jacket ventilators, which enclose only the thorax and abdomen, have been developed but they are less efficient.[3] Optimal sealing of the cuirass, with adequate room for expansion, is best achieved by making a custombuilt shell for each patient but leakage and friction at pressure points may still be a problem.[4] Discomfort has been a major reason for withdrawal from studies of negative pressure ventilation in patients with COPD.[5-7]

A small number of patients who are unable to breathe adequately at any time (for example following high cervical cord injury) require continuous ventilatory assistance. This is best provided by tracheostomy and positive pressure ventilation or, occasionally, by diaphragmatic pacing.[8] A battery power source allows some mobility, though the constraints of size limit this to a few hours. Ventilator malfunction or power failure can be catastrophic and suitable arrangements must be made to cater for this possibility. If aspiration of pharyngeal secretions is a problem a cuffed tube is necessary, however the system is closed and spontaneous breaths are not possible in the event of ventilator failure or incoordination between the patient's respiratory efforts and machine imposed breaths. The cuff must be deflated or a speaking tube inserted by day, to permit speech. The major disadvantage is the morbidity and occasional mortality associated with tracheostomy.[9]

Rationale for assisted ventilation during sleep

When ventilation is assisted during sleep, most patients requiring domiciliary ventilation can be kept in good health, often for many years, with improved daytime symptoms and arterial blood gas tensions.[10-13] At first, improvement during the day following assisted ventilation during sleep seems surprising. However, profound abnormalities of gas exchange can occur during sleep in patients with neuromuscular disorders and chest wall deformity, even when they are relatively well by day[14] (figure 5.1). Repeated episodes of hypoxaemia and hypercapnia during sleep lead, in time, to the development of daytime respiratory failure, pulmonary hypertension, right heart failure and death.[15]

Wakefulness is an important stimulus to breathe and mild hypoventilation during sleep,[16 17] with an increment in carbon dioxide tension of up to 6 mm Hg is normal. However, in patients with little respiratory reserve marked oxygen desaturation and hypercapnia can occur. The respiratory reserve is reduced in scoliosis because the work of breathing is increased by deformity and rigidity of the chest wall and reduced lung compliance.[18] Rapid eye movement (REM) sleep may be associated with severe hypoxaemia and worsening hypercapnia,[14] because during this phase

81

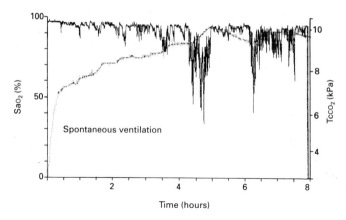

FIG 5.1—Levels of arterial oxygen saturation and transcutaneous carbon dioxide in a 19-year-old patient with Duchenne muscular dystrophy presenting with morning headaches and nausea on waking. Daytime arterial blood gas tensions measured at 17.00 hours were: Pao_2 12.5 kPa, $Paco_2$ 5.4 kPa, BE 4.3 mmol/l. Nocturnal study shows marked desaturation and severe progressive rise in transcutaneous CO_2 despite relatively normal values at the start of the night.

of sleep there is a profound loss of postural muscle activity and ventilation is largely dependent on diaphragm function.[19] Diaphragm contractility may be impaired: as part of a primary neuromuscular disease; by poor perfusion; by hypoxia and hypercapnia; through inadequate ventilation; or its action may be compromised because of working at a mechanical disadvantage as a consequence of an abnormal chest configuration.[20 21] In patients who are mainly dependent on accessory muscles, the diaphragm alone is unable to maintain ventilation during REM sleep and marked oxygen desaturation and hypercapnia occur.

The effectiveness of assisted ventilation in patients unable to maintain adequate ventilation because of an inadequate respiratory muscle pump is not surprising. A logical case can also be made for the extension of this technique to patients with lung disease associated with a degree of alveolar hypoventilation and most work has been done in COPD. These patients, particularly those who are hypercapnic by day, hypoventilate during sleep and this is particularly marked during REM sleep.[22-24] Renal retention of bicarbonate ions occurs to buffer the acidosis following transient increases in $Paco_2$ leading to a reduction in central ventilatory drive. Finally the respiratory muscles are at a mechanical disadvantage because of hyperinflation.[25] This has led to the proposal that ventilatory failure occurs, in part, because of chronic fatigue of the respiratory muscles which should improve if respiratory muscles are given the opportunity to "rest".[26]

Choice of equipment

Almost any ventilator can be used for nasal ventilation. Most modern ventilators, used in intensive care units are unnecessarily sophisticated and therefore too expensive for widespread domiciliary use.

There is often confusion between NPPV and CPAP, because both can be used with a nasal mask and both are used at home for sleep related disturbances of breathing. However CPAP is only effective if the patient is breathing spontaneously and it cannot provide ventilation if the patient becomes apnoeic. When CPAP is used with a nasal mask, low pressures of 5–15 cm H_2O, are effective in splinting the upper airway and preventing upper airway obstruction in patients with obstructive sleep apnoea (OSA).[27] It can also be used to improve gas exchange in patients with lung disease, particularly interstitial disorders.[28-30] It is thought to recruit collapsed alveoli and reduces the work of breathing by increasing the FRC, thus moving the patient onto a more beneficial part of the pressure–volume curve. In patients with severe COPD it reduces respiratory effort by counterbalancing the inspiratory threshold load imposed by intrinsic $PEEP_i$.[31-33]

The ventilators used for NPPV fall into two broad categories, volume cycled flow generators (VCFG) and pressure cycled flow generators. A number of different ventilators, with slightly different features, are available (table 5.1). With VCFGs a fixed tidal volume is delivered and to achieve this the inflation pressure may vary from breath to breath. The ventilator should be capable of generating high pressures and delivering large minute volumes. This is important when the nasal route is used, because tidal volumes up to twice those used in intubated patients are necessary to compensate for leaks around the mask and through the mouth and to ventilate the increased deadspace of the nasopharynx. If there are no spontaneous inspiratory efforts or they are too feeble to trigger the ventilator, an automatic cycle must be imposed to ensure that gas exchange continues. A sensitive trigger with a short

TABLE 5.1—Commonly used ventilators in the United Kingdom

Volume cycled flow generators	
The Brompton Pac	Pneupac Ltd, Crescent Road, Luton, Beds LU2 0AH (Telephone 0582 445303)
Monnal D	Deva Medical Electronics Ltd, 8 Jensen Court, Astmore Industrial Estate, Runcorn, Cheshire WA7 1SQ (Telephone 09285 65836)
PLV Lifecare	Lifecare GMBH, Hauptstrasse 60, D-8031 Seefeld 2, Germany (Telephone 010 49 8152 79669)
Pressure cycled flow generators	
The BiPAP	Medicaid Ltd, Hook Lane, Pagham, Sussex PO21 3PP (Telephone 0243 268718)
The Nippy	Thomas Respiratory Systems, 33 Half Moon Lane, Herne Hill, London SE24 9JX (Telephone 071 737 5881)

response time is necessary if the work of breathing is not to be increased during triggered ventilation.[34] Where there is a choice (for example with the PLV Lifecare system) the assist–control mode ensures that breaths are triggered or imposed depending on the presence and magnitude of the inspiratory efforts of the patient.

Pressure limited devices deliver a predetermined pressure and therefore the tidal volume may vary from breath to breath, particularly in patients with a changing impedance to inflation. These devices can be subdivided into those in which the predetermined pressure is maintained throughout inspiration (for example the BiPAP and the Nippy) and those in which the machine cycles into expiration as soon as that pressure is reached (for example the Bird (M and IE Dentsply, Sowton Industrial Estate, Exeter) and the Bennett (UK supplier: Puritan Bennett, 152–176 Great South West Road, Hounslow, Middlesex)). The BiPAP and Nippy are variable flow generators which can increase flow to compensate for leaks from around the mask and through the open mouth. When triggered they effectively provide pressure support ventilation, but can provide full ventilation in the event of apnoea. They are relatively small, easily portable and require little maintenance.

A number of different BiPAP models are available, but most patients require one which can be used in the spontaneous/triggered mode. During spontaneous breathing the machine triggers on changes in flow and effectively provides pressure support. A minimum respiratory rate can be set so that the machine automatically cycles into inspiration in the event of apnoea. The level of expiratory

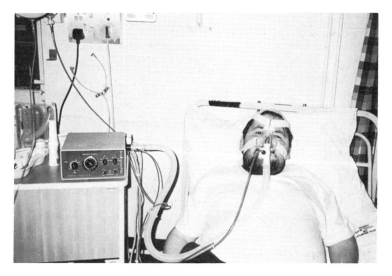

FIG 5.2—Patient receiving nasal ventilation.

positive airway pressure can be adjusted and may be of benefit in some patients with neuromuscular and skeletal disorders or COPD.

The Bird and the Bennett Systems can be used to augment spontaneous ventilation. Gas flow from the machine ceases when a predetermined pressure is reached, and the expiratory pathway is then open to the atmosphere. Because inspiration is terminated when a preset pressure is reached the tidal volume may be insufficient particularly when the impedance to inflation is high. Their main use is as physiotherapy aids, to re-expand atelectatic lungs or for the administration of nebulised bronchodilators.

The patient–ventilator interface

The ventilator is connected to the patient via tubing and a mask, which is held in position over the nose by a series of straps (figure 5.2). It can be applied and removed by the patient, though those with weak upper limbs may require some assistance. The mask may need to be applied quite tightly to the face to maintain a good seal, leading to some soreness, particularly over the bridge of the nose. Most patients quickly get used to this and it does not usually cause difficulties during long term domiciliary use. However pressure damage may be a problem when patients are ventilated for much of the day. Excessive soreness and tissue breakdown can be prevented by the use of sticking plaster or other cushioning material over pressure areas. The barrier material used to protect the skin round abdominal stomata (for example Granuflex) can also be helpful. Pressure on the bridge of the nose can be minimised by using a soft wedge to lift the apex of the mask away from the face. With modern silicone masks, which have a deep flange, leaks can often be reduced by slackening, rather than tightening, the head straps thereby allowing the flanges to flatten against the face. A vicious cycle sometimes develops with the patient or carer pulling the mask tighter and tighter against the face, with increasing leakage and discomfort.

A wide range of commercially manufactured masks is now available and an adequate seal can usually be achieved, but occasionally custombuilt masks may be necessary. Soft plastic plugs (the Adams circuit) inserted into the nares, shaped so that the delivery of positive pressure through the lumen helps seal the wall of the plug against the inner surface of the nasal vestibule, may be more effective or better tolerated in some patients.[35][36] This technique may be particularly useful as a means of protecting the nasal bridge in patients requiring NPPV for much of the day, for instance during infective exacerbations. Leaks from the mouth, particularly during sleep, can be reduced by a chin strap.

Initiating NPPV

The patient should be acclimatised to the system in hospital with medical and nursing staff familiar with the technique readily available. A successful outcome is less likely if NPPV is attempted on a ward without the necessary expertise. Very breathless patients may need to start NPPV sitting up, but in most it is preferable if they are lying back in bed at about 45 degrees, or alternatively in an easy chair. When possible the patient should first be allowed to hold the mask in position over the nose for a few trial breaths. While this is usually associated with a very poor seal and a large leak around the mask, it allows the patient to experience the sensation of nasal positive pressure. Once the patient has gained confidence the head gear can be assembled and the mask held in place more securely. Small tidal volumes should be used initially, to avoid a sudden surge of pressure which may be very uncomfortable. The patient can then be encouraged to help determine the ventilator settings for respiratory rate, the length of inspiration and the size of breaths. As the patient acclimatises to the system, accessory muscle activity is reduced and the patient often drifts off to sleep. Before being left alone, the patient should be shown how to disconnect the ventilator tubing from the mask and told what to do in the event of the ventilator alarm sounding.

Pulse oximetry may be helpful initially, particularly in severely ill patients, and the levels of arterial blood gas tensions should be checked after approximately 30–40 minutes and subsequently, to ensure adequate control of hypercapnia. The $PaCO_2$ is often unchanged initially, but gradually reduces over the next few hours. In severely ill patients it is best to add oxygen from the outset, usually via a port in the nasal mask, at a flow rate of 1–2 l/min.

Patients using the ventilator should be encouraged to sleep as soon as possible and at this stage the low pressure alarm, which detects appreciable leaks, need not be set with particular stringency, except for patients particularly vulnerable to even small reductions in minute volume. Once the patient is able to sleep for much of the night the low pressure alarm should be set, usually to a value of about 10–15 cm H_2O less than peak inflation pressure, so that appreciable leaks are detected. The usual source of inadvertent volume loss is from leaks around the mask or through the mouth in those who sleep with their mouth open. This can be reduced by using an elasticated chin strap. Edentulous patients should be encouraged to retain their dentures. Sometimes a full face mask is required. Other sources of gas leak should be sought if the low pressure alarm sounds and there is no evidence of leakage around the mask or through the mouth. All connections, and the integrity of the tubing and mask, should be checked. Dislodgement of the caps, which cover the ports in the mask is a common occurrence.

Most volume cycled machines are equipped with a high pressure alarm and/or pneumatic cut out. This may activate occasionally during normal use in patients when the impedance to inflation increases, for example, if the patient is trying to talk or moving around. More frequent activation raises the possibility of upper airway obstruction. This can usually be corrected by encouraging the patient to lean back on pillows, thereby slightly extending the neck. If the high pressure alarm continues to sound without obvious explanation, disconnect the tubing from the mask. The inflation pressure should fall to less than 10 cm H_2O; if it does not there is increased resistance from the tubing, usually because of a faulty valve, which should be replaced. A faulty expiratory valve should be suspected when positive pressure registers on the pressure dial during expiration (unless of course PEEP or EPAP has been added).

In the acute situation some severely dyspnoeic patients breathe through the mouth. As well as promoting leaks, this effectively bypasses the ventilator, which is therefore not triggered in response to the patient's efforts and marked asynchrony occurs. This is very inefficient and uncomfortable for the patient. In such circumstances full face mask ventilation may be successful. However the circuit is now closed and close supervision is therefore necessary in case of ventilator failure.

Occasionally patients complain of rhinorrhoea or excessive nasal dryness, which can be helped by ipratropium bromide nasal drops or humidification, respectively. For humidification, the insertion of a simple heat and moisture exchanger into the circuit may be sufficient. However these devices may increase the work of breathing during assisted breaths and should probably be changed daily, which greatly increases the cost. If necessary a humidifier can be incorporated into the ventilator circuit. Nasal blockage may be a problem, particularly during an upper respiratory tract infection and can be helped by the short term use of ephedrine nasal drops.

Gaseous distension may be troublesome, particularly when the impedance to inflation is high or the patient breathes out of synchrony with the ventilator. It can be reduced by using the assist-control mode and by minimising peak inflation pressure. There should be a low threshold for passing a nasogastric tube, even though this will interfere with the seal between the mask and the face, if abdominal distension occurs when a full face mask is used. This is because of the substantial risk of aspiration should the patient vomit into the mask.

If patients are to be sent home the adequacy of ventilation during sleep should be confirmed (figure 5.3). Arterial blood gas tensions measured with NPPV during wakefulness may be misleading because the mouth is more firmly closed and at least some respiratory effort augments ventilation. Continuous measurement of $EtCO_2$ or $PtcCO_2$ is advisable because quite substantial reductions in ventilation may pass unnoticed if only oxygen saturation is recorded. A checklist for initiating NPPV is given in table 5.2.

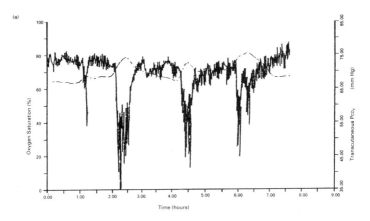

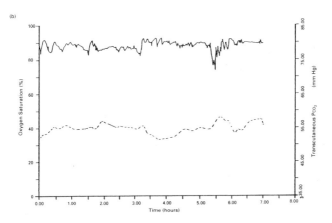

FIG 5.3—Overnight studies of oxygen saturation (solid line) and transcutaneous carbon dioxide (broken line) in a patient with kyphoscoliosis and mild COPD. (a) Breathing air spontaneously. Note the low baseline saturation at the start of the night and the episodes of profound desaturation associated with a rise in the $TcCo_2$ (b) With NPPV.

Patient selection

Chest wall disorders and stable neuromuscular disease

The chief indication for NPPV is hypercapnic respiratory failure which has failed to respond to maximal conventional treatment. Worldwide the largest group of patients receiving domiciliary NPPV consists of those with chest wall disorders and/or non-progressive neuromuscular disease.

89

TABLE 5.2—Initiating NPPV

- In hospital
- Ready access to experienced nursing and medical staff
- Start with small tidal volumes
- Add oxygen from the outset in the severely ill
- Check arterial blood gas tensions after 30–60 minutes
- Encourage use of chin strap if appreciable mouth leak
- Low threshold for nasogastric tube if abdominal distension while using full face mask
- Check adequacy of ventilation during sleep if patient to take ventilator home
- If alarms sound
  Low pressure
    Check mask position
    Encourage use of chin strap
    Check connectors, tubing and mask
  High pressure
    ?Neck flexed and upper airway obstructed
    ?Obstruction in tubing

The selection of patients for elective treatment with NPPV, depends on the accurate recognition of high risk groups, and suitable assessment and monitoring of ventilatory function. Patient groups at risk of developing hypercapnic ventilatory failure are listed in table 5.3.

Thoracic scoliosis is idiopathic in 80% of patients, with the spinal curvature developing typically at the time of the adolescent growth spurt. Scoliosis can also occur in neuromuscular disease, inherited disorders such as neurofibromatosis and Marfan's syndrome and following chest wall surgery. Respiratory insufficiency occurring later in life is rare in patients with an adolescent-onset idiopathic deformity, unless there is additional cardiac or respiratory pathology. However, up to 70% of individuals who acquire a scoliosis before the age of 5 years develop cardiorespiratory problems as a consequence of their chest wall disease.[37] A vital capacity at presentation of less than 50% predicted should indicate the need for long term follow-up. A high thoracic curvature appears to place the respiratory muscles (including accessory muscles) at a greater mechanical disadvantage than a low thoracic scoliosis. The severity of the curvature is an obvious risk factor in idiopathic scoliosis, but there is little correlation between the degree of curvature and respiratory function in patients with neuromuscular disorders.

TABLE 5.3—Patients with the following disorders are at risk of developing ventilatory failure

Chest wall disorders
Early onset idiopathic scoliosis
Thoracoplasty
Rigid spine syndrome
Fibrothorax

Primary muscle disorders
Congenital and acquired myopathies (for example acid maltase deficiency, mitochondrial myopathy, central core disease)
Muscular dystrophies (for example Duchenne, congenital, fascio–scapular–humeral, Becker)
Myotonic dystrophy

Neuromuscular junction
Myasthenia gravis

Disorders of the spinal cord and peripheral nerves
Poliomyelitis
Spinal muscular atrophy
Motor neurone disease
High (cervical) spinal cord lesions
Phrenic nerve lesions
Polyneuropathies (congenital and acquired)

Central disorders
Brainstem lesions
Hypothalamic disorders
Primary alveolar hypoventilation
Central sleep apnoea
Encephalitis

Studies of nocturnal respiration in neuromuscular disease have shown that the minimum arterial oxygen saturation level during sleep is correlated with vital capacity and the percentage fall in vital capacity when changing from an erect to a supine position.[38] A fall in vital capacity when supine indicates significant diaphragm weakness. Measurement of respiratory muscle strength can also be a helpful way of monitoring patients. Braun[39] has demonstrated that in a group of patients with neuromuscular disorders, a maximal inspiratory mouth pressure of less than 30% predicted is associated with daytime hypercapnia.

Chest wall disease may complicate the picture in other situations. For example, hypercapnic respiratory failure in a patient with previous tuberculosis may be the result of extra pulmonary restriction caused by a thoracoplasty and phrenic nerve crush, pulmonary restriction as a consequence of post-tuberculous lung fibrosis and chronic airflow obstruction due to lung disease related to smoking.

In all patients with chest wall disease and neuromuscular disorders a vital capacity of less than 1 litre places the individual at risk of developing ventilatory failure. These patients should be questioned specifically about the presence of symptoms of nocturnal hypoventilation, as these features can develop insidiously and may be attributed by the patient simply to ageing. Assessment of full pulmonary function will allow independently treatable conditions such as chronic airflow obstruction to be addressed, and enable the physician to follow serial changes in lung function. A progressive fall in vital capacity and total lung capacity usually heralds the onset of respiratory insufficiency in restrictive chest wall disease.

The measurement of arterial blood gas tensions is mandatory when nocturnal hypoventilation is suspected. The presence of an elevated base excess or daytime hypercapnia is an indication for nocturnal monitoring of arterial oxygen saturation and, ideally, transcutaneous $Paco_2$ and respiratory effort during sleep. As a guide, a peak nocturnal $Paco_2$ of more than 8 kPa and an Sao_2 value of less than 90% for most of the night, when accompanied by symptoms of hypoventilation, are taken as indications for starting NPPV. Occasionally patients may be helped by medical treatment such as protriptyline (a non-sedating tricyclic antidepressant) used in doses of 10–20 mg at night, which suppresses rapid eye movement sleep and has been shown to improve symptoms and diurnal arterial blood gas tensions.[40 41] Intermittent courses of NPPV in hospital may also be helpful. Long term oxygen therapy (LTOT) is usually contraindicated in chest wall disease associated with ventilatory failure as it provokes unacceptable carbon dioxide retention in all but a handful of patients with severe restriction.

The adequacy of ventilation during NPPV should be confirmed once the patient has become acclimatised to nocturnal ventilatory support, by monitoring Sao_2 and $Ptcco_2$. Outpatient follow-up should include a regular check of arterial blood gas tensions and lung function.

Outcome of domiciliary NPPV   Over the last decade, information has emerged on the outcome of NPPV in patients with chest wall and stable or slowly progressive neuromuscular disease. There have been no controlled trials, but French and British studies of patients receiving nocturnal support[42 43] have demonstrated convincing benefit with a 5 year survival rate of around 85% in early onset scoliosis and up to 100% in post polio patients. In the studies, arterial blood gas tensions were maintained and the patient's quality of life was generally well preserved.

Progressive neuromuscular disease Until recently, the question of ventilatory support in rapidly progressive neuromuscular disorders, such as motor neurone disease, was never raised. In many patients with these conditions death occurs from respiratory complications. In most individuals respiratory support is inappropriate and only adds to the burden of the illness. However, NPPV can be considered to treat symptoms of breathlessness and nocturnal hypoventilation in patients with early respiratory muscle involvement and preserved general muscle strength, and to help patients who have presented in respiratory failure and require intubation before a diagnosis is reached. Any decision to implement ventilatory support needs to take into account the wishes of the patient and family, and the practical problems likely to be faced by all concerned. Assisted ventilation in Duchenne muscular dystrophy is discussed below.

Lung disease
A number of studies have shown that it is possible to ventilate patients with intrinsic lung disease, particularly COPD, at home using NPPV.[11 44-46] Successful NPPV results in an improvement in arterial blood gas tensions during spontaneous breathing by day (figure 5.4), better quality of sleep and improved exercise capacity. However, domiciliary oxygen therapy is the current "gold standard" for the treatment of respiratory failure due to COPD. It has been shown to improve survival,[47 48] but though compliance was very good in the trials this is not always the case in routine clinical practice, the main reason being the restriction placed on lifestyle by the need for 16 hours of oxygen per day.[49 50] The failure to control hypercapnia, which appears to be associated with a worse prognosis,[48 51 52] is a further problem with LTOT. These limitations suggest that NPPV during sleep, which does not interfere with daytime activities and reduces CO_2 tension, may be better tolerated and improve survival in COPD. It is relevant to note, however,

(a)

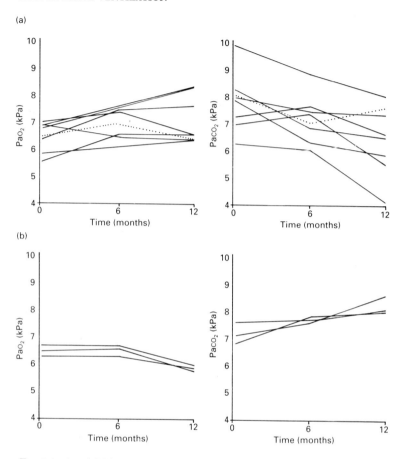

(b)

FIG 5.4—Arterial blood gas tensions during spontaneous breathing in the mid afternoon before starting nasal intermittent positive pressure ventilation and after 6 and 12 months. (a) Seven patients still using ventilation at home at 12 months (solid lines) and one patient (case 4) who discontinued ventilation after 9 months (broken line). (b) Three patients who discontinued home ventilation before 6 months. Taken from Elliott et al.[46]

that oxygen given only overnight was associated with a worse survival rate than when given continuously in the NOTT study.[47] The place of NPPV in the management of chronic respiratory failure in COPD can only be determined by a large scale randomised comparison with domiciliary oxygen therapy; a multi-centre European trial is currently in progress.

TABLE 5.4—Domiciliary NPPV in COPD

- Patient deteriorating despite maximum conventional treatment
- Hypercapnia
- Not endstage emphysema
- Motivation
- In patient acclimatisation and education
- Documented nocturnal hypoventilation breathing spontaneously
- Documented control of nocturnal hypoventilation by NPPV
- A 6 month trial if tolerated

Although it cannot currently be recommended as first line treatment for hypercapnic patients with COPD, a trial of NPPV should be considered in those patients who deteriorate despite oxygen therapy or who are intolerant of it (table 5.4). Well motivated hypercapnic patients are most likely to benefit from NPPV and adequate education and acclimatisation to the technique are essential. Initiation of ventilation in hospital is preferable, though more costly, and the adequacy of control of nocturnal hypoventilation needs to be confirmed. Muir[53] has suggested increasing treatment as the disease progresses, starting with oxygen given through a mask or nasal cannulae and if this is inadequate transtracheally. If this fails, NPPV is added and finally positive pressure ventilation via tracheostomy is considered.

The use of NPPV has also been described in cystic fibrosis and other types of bronchiectasis. It has been used as a "bridge to transplantation" in patients with cystic fibrosis.[54] with a better eventual outcome than in those who required intubation and ventilation.[54 55] It has the additional advantages that the patients are able to cooperate with physiotherapy, be involved in discussions about their management and can maintain nutrition and a degree of mobility. They can be managed on a general medical ward, rather than in an intensive care unit, which is more pleasant for the patients and their relatives and is considerably less expensive. However, because of the success of heart and heart/lung transplantation more patients have been considered for the operation and waiting lists have grown. Sadly many patients do not receive a transplant, though they can be kept alive for up to 29 months.[56] With such prolonged waiting times patients become increasingly dependent on the ventilator. NPPV provides symptomatic relief of dyspnoea, but skin breakdown over the nasal bridge may be a problem.

Generally domiciliary assisted ventilation for patients with bronchiectasis is associated with a much worse outcome than for other patient groups.[43][57] However Leger et al[58] have reported better results with an actuarial probability of continuing NPPV at 5 years of 62% in 25 patients with bronchiectasis. This compares favourably with sequelae of tuberculosis (60%), Duchenne muscular dystrophy (47%) and COPD (31%).

Children

Home ventilation can be used in children who develop hypercapnic respiratory failure as a consequence of conditions such as congenital or acquired myopathy, muscular dystrophy, chest wall disease and the alveolar hypoventilation syndromes. Up to the age of 2 years, positive pressure ventilation via a tracheostomy is usually required, especially if the child is heavily dependent on the ventilator and/ or bulbar reflexes are impaired. Early reports of NPPV suggested that it was impossible to apply nasal masks or face masks successfully in children below the age of 6 years. However, recent experience has shown that they can be used effectively in some children as young as 2 years of age.[59] Negative pressure delivered by portable mini iron lungs and jacket devices can also work well in this group.

Duchenne's muscular dystrophy (DMD) is the most common form of muscular dystrophy, with an incidence of 1:5000 male births. In most cases motor delay is evident by the age of 3 years and the majority of affected children are wheelchair-bound by 12 years. A progressive loss of lung function is seen from adolescence onwards, with death occurring from respiratory failure or cardiac complications between the age of 20 and 25 years. The extent of respiratory muscle involvement tends to reflect the degree of peripheral muscle weakness. Use of assisted ventilation in DMD is a controversial issue. Its use during the early asymptomatic stage of the disease, and late in the course of the disease should be distinguished. Some workers have advocated ventilatory assistance before nocturnal symptoms have developed, to prevent progression to respiratory failure. There is no evidence to support intervention at this point; it may be harmful, and is certainly burdensome to patients. In contrast, clinical experience strongly suggests that nocturnal non-invasive ventilation can be of value in selected patients with prominent symptoms of nocturnal hypoventilation (especially morning headaches, disturbed sleep, breathlessness and fatigue) and documented nocturnal hypercapnia.

It is not clear which is the best ventilatory support method in DMD. Monitoring respiratory disturbances during sleep has shown that obstructive apnoeas and hypopnoeas may occur in addition to central hypoventilation. This is likely to be due to pharyngeal muscle dysfunction. Any tendency to upper airway collapse during sleep may be exacerbated by negative pressure ventilation,[60] suggesting that NPPV may be preferable to negative pressure methods; trials comparing the two methods are underway. As the disease progresses patients inevitably become more dependent on the ventilator. Most do not elect to undergo tracheostomy when aspiration and other bulbar symptoms become a problem. It is important that these issues are carefully explored with patients and their families, at the time ventilatory support is initiated.

The burden of caring for a child or adolescent dependent on a ventilator should not be underestimated. Full community and hospital support should be available to families, including the facility for respite admissions.

Mechanisms of improvement in daytime function

The mechanism by which NPPV used during sleep improves daytime function and arterial blood gas tensions is multifactorial and controversial. It is helpful to consider the effects of assisted ventilation on subsequent spontaneous ventilation in terms of the capacity of the system, the load on it and the central drive to breathe. An improvement may therefore occur if capacity or central drive increase or load is reduced.

Improved capacity

One difficulty in exploring this hypothesis is the lack of any objective test of chronic fatigue. Some studies of non-invasive ventilation have cited increased respiratory muscle strength as evidence of the resolution of chronic fatigue.[44 61-63] However, tests of respiratory muscle strength require maximum voluntary efforts by the patients and an improvement in general well being may have been responsible for the enhanced performance. Others have reported successful control of chronic ventilatory failure, but without increased respiratory muscle strength.[1][64][65] Shapiro *et al*[7] attempted to reduce respiratory muscle EMG activity using negative pressure devices in a randomised placebo controlled study. While this was not uniformly successful there was no evidence that respiratory muscle rest was of benefit.

Restored chemosensitivity

Improved chemosensitivity following the control of nocturnal hypoventilation has been shown in patients with OSA[66] and COPD.[65] Goldstein and coworkers[10] showed that non-invasive ventilation in patients with neuromuscular disease reduced the severity of night time hypercapnia if ventilatory support was subsequently omitted, suggesting an increased central sensitivity to CO_2.

Reduced load

Some studies have demonstrated an increase in vital capacity after prolonged treatment.[12][18][67] The mechanism of increase in vital capacity in these studies could be an improvement in pulmonary compliance consequent upon reversal of small airway closure and microatelectasis or perhaps reduced stiffness of the bony rib cage and soft tissues of the chest wall. Other studies have not shown this,[1][10][64] and in most circumstances it is likely that any reduction in ventilatory load secondary to improved compliance is a relatively minor factor in the reversal of ventilatory failure.

Current evidence suggests that the pivotal action of NPPV in reversing chronic ventilatory failure is its capacity to control nocturnal hypoventilation. It is possible that the efficiency of NPPV, whether it provides all or only part of ventilation, whether the respiratory muscles are "rested" or not is of no great importance as long as nocturnal hypoventilation is controlled. Similarly the particular technique of non-invasive ventilation may be largely irrelevant provided that the method used controls nocturnal hypoxaemia and hypercapnia.

Acute on chronic ventilatory failure

The widespread use of NPPV in the management of chronic ventilatory failure has encouraged its use in selected patients with acute ventilatory failure. Although non-invasive ventilation using negative pressure by tank ventilators[68] and positive pressure by mouth piece[69] were tried 30 years ago, endotracheal intubation and ventilation have been the mainstay of management for acute ventilatory failure. NPPV has now become a treatment option for some patients who would otherwise be managed by intubation, or perhaps would not be mechanically ventilated at all. As an alternative to intubation, NPPV has many advantages. Without the need for sedation, patients can be alert and communicative, can swallow and achieve a level of control and independence totally different from when intubated. The use of the technique in the treatment of acute ventilatory failure has been described in COPD[45 70-78] chest wall disorders,[45 72 73 75 77] pneumonia,[70 74 77] cardiac failure,[70 74 77] cystic fibrosis,[56 79] OSA[80] and postoperatively.[74]

Chest wall disorders

Many patients are now successfully managed with domiciliary nasal ventilation used only during sleep. When they develop an additional problem, for example pulmonary infection, it is often necessary to increase the duration of NPPV. "Acute exacerbations" are therefore easily managed by NPPV in this patient group. Similarly there are a number of patients with severe chest wall disorders, particularly kyphoscoliosis, who do not require NPPV on a regular basis, but do require such treatment from time to time when additional problems arise.

COPD

The situation in patients with copd is less clear cut and there are few data from controlled studies. Recommendations for the use of domiciliary nasal positive pressure ventilation are given in table 5.4. Brochard and coworkers[71] used inspiratory pressure support via full face mask for an average of 7 hours each day for between 2 and 6 days in 13 patients with acute exacerbations of COPD, who they judged would probably have needed intubation. Only one of their patients needed intubation compared with eleven of thirteen patients in a historical control group. The study patients also spent less time in the intensive care unit. More recently, Bott and colleagues[78] have performed a prospective randomised clinical trial of NPPV compared with conventional therapy in patients with acute exacerbations of COPD characterised by hypoxia and hypercapnia. Thirty patients were randomised to receive NPPV and 30 patients received conventional therapy. Nasal ventilation was more effective than conventional therapy in lowering $PaCO_2$ and reversing acidosis. Nine of 30 patients died in the conventionally treated group and three of 30 patients in the NPPV group. This difference was not quite statistically significant ($p = 0.1$) when analysed on an intention to treat basis. Four patients allocated to have NPPV did not receive it; one patient had a chronic nose injury which made it impossible, one patient refused all therapy, and two patients were confused and uncooperative (one of whom died). A comparison of the 26 patients who were treated with NPPV with the 30 patients who received conventional therapy demonstrated a significant reduction in mortality ($p = 0.01$).

These results, plus those documented in a number of descriptive studies, support the use of NPPV in patients with COPD and acute respiratory failure who for whatever reason are not suitable for endotracheal intubation and positive pressure ventilation. In those deemed suitable for intubation, NPPV can be tried first and if it fails the patient can then be intubated. If necessary NPPV can be used subsequently to help wean the patient.

Weaning from conventional ventilation

Weaning problems occur in up to 20% of patients who receive IPPV. The overall figure is dependent on the nature of the acute event requiring ventilatory assistance, the period of time spent on the ventilator, and the general condition of the patient.[81] It is a familiar observation in intensive care units that the majority of individuals who develop weaning difficulties have significant underlying respiratory, cardiac or neuromuscular pathology. Bearing in mind the precarious balance between ventilatory capacity and demand that exists at rest in patients with severe cardiorespiratory or neuromuscular disease, it is not surprising that they are unable to sustain the increase in cardiorespiratory workload which is needed during the transition from IPPV to spontaneous breathing.

Weaning problems can be circumvented by using NPPV to treat acute hypercapnic exacerbations of chronic lung disease as described above, thereby avoiding intubation and admission to the intensive care unit. However, some patients continue to receive IPPV after elective or emergency surgery, and others may be intubated to aid the clearance of bronchial secretions. Before the weaning process begins remediable causes of respiratory failure should be addressed,[82] and pulmonary and cardiac function optimised. Patients are likely to benefit from a gradual withdrawal of respiratory support using ventilatory modes such as pressure sup-

TABLE 5.5—Criteria for weaning using NPPV

- Normal bulbar function
- Able to breathe spontaneously for at least 5 minutes
- Minimal sputum production
- Low requirement for supplemental oxygen
- Stable haemodynamic status
- Functioning gastrointestinal tract

---

port or intermittent mandatory ventilation. Where these strategies fail NPPV can prove a useful alternative and should be considered before carrying out a tracheostomy. Candidates suitable for weaning using NPPV should meet the criteria listed in table 5.5.

As NPPV does not secure control of the airway, normal bulbar function including an adequate cough reflex is an essential requirement. Patients should also have a functioning gastrointestinal tract, because if an ileus is present NPPV can provoke troublesome gastric distension. It is important that the patient should be able to breathe spontaneously for at least 5 minutes before transfer to NPPV is attempted so that sufficient time is allowed for fitting and adjustment of the mask.

Alert and cooperative patients with an endotracheal tube in situ can be extubated and transferred straight on to mask ventilation. A trial of NPPV is *not* contraindicated in the presence of tracheostomy,[83] but the tracheostomy track should be well established to reduce the risk of subcutaneous emphysema. In most patients, NPPV is continued at first for about 16–20 hours a day, including nocturnal use. Patients can be transferred from the intensive care unit to a general ward if staff experience allows. It is usually possible gradually to reduce the amount of time spent receiving ventilatory support depending on diurnal and nocturnal arterial blood gas measurements. In a study[84] of patients with chronic respiratory, cardiorespiratory or neuromuscular disease who had failed standard trials of weaning, about 80% were successfully established on NPPV (figure 5.5). Some patients with extensive pulmonary fibrosis who were unable to tolerate the ventilatory pattern of the nasal ventilator failed to respond. This is not unexpected as the performance characteristics of volume and pressure preset nasal ventilators are unlikely to meet the complex ventilatory requirements of patients with end stage interstitial lung disease.

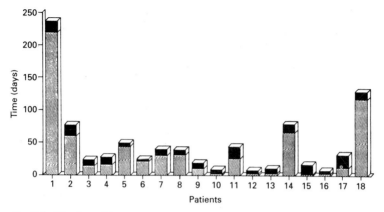

FIG 5.5—Number of days patients received conventional ventilation (hatched area) and the number of days from the start of NPPV (dark area) until hospital discharge. Taken from Udwadia et al.[84]

A proportion of patients weaned successfully by NPPV, particularly those with chest wall and neuromuscular disorders, may require long term domiciliary ventilatory support at night.[84][85] The decision to provide such support should be based on diurnal and nocturnal arterial blood gas control, the overall prognosis, and the wishes of the patient and family.

Conclusion

The option of assisting ventilation non-invasively in patients with acute on chronic ventilatory failure is a useful addition to the therapeutic armamentarium of respiratory physicians and intensivists. The use of positive pressure delivered via nasal or face mask has greatly widened the applicability of non-invasive ventilation, because it can be achieved in most hospitals using existing machines, with only a little extra expenditure for masks and head gear. However patients thought to require domiciliary ventilation should be managed by centres with experience in this specialised area of respiratory care.

1 Mohr CH, Hill NS. Long-term follow-up of nocturnal ventilatory assistance in patients with respiratory failure due to Duchenne-type muscular dystrophy. *Chest* 1990;**97**:91–6.
2 Ellis ER, Bye PTB, Bruderer JW, Sullivan CE. Treatment of respiratory failure during sleep in patients with neuromuscular disease. *Am Rev Respir Dis* 1987;**135**:148–52.
3 Kinnear WJM, Shneerson JM. Assisted ventilation at home: is it worth considering? *Br J Dis Chest* 1985;**79**:313–51.

4 Brown L, Kinnear WJM, Sergeant KA *et al.* Artificial ventilation by external negative pressure – a method for making cuirass shells. *Physiotherapy* 1985;**71**:181–3.
5 Zibrak JD, Hill NS, Federman EC, Kwa SL, O'Donnell C. Evaluation of intermittent long term negative-pressure ventilation in patients with severe COPD. *Am Rev Respir Dis* 1988;**138**:1515–18.
6 Celli B, Lee H, Criner G *et al.* Controlled trial of external negative pressure ventilation in patients with severe chronic airflow limitation. *Am Rev Respir Dis* 1989;**140**:1251–6.
7 Shapiro SH, Ernst P, Gray-Donald K *et al.* Effect of negative pressure ventilation in severe chronic obstructive pulmonary disease. *Lancet* 1992;**340**:1425–9.
8 Moxham J, Shneerson JM. Diaphragmatic pacing. *Am Rev Respir Dis* 1993;**148**:533–6.
9 Stauffer JL, Olson DE, Petty TL. Complications and consequences of endotracheal intubation and tracheostomy. *Am J Med* 1981;**70**:65–75.
10 Goldstein RS, Molotiu N, Skrastins R *et al.* Reversal of sleep-induced hypoventilation and chronic respiratory failure by nocturnal negative pressure ventilation in patients with restrictive ventilatory impairment. *Am Rev Respir Dis* 1987;**135**:1049–55.
11 Carroll N, Branthwaite MA. Control of nocturnal hypoventilation by nasal intermittent positive pressure ventilation. *Thorax* 1988;**43**:349–53.
12 Hoeppner VH, Cockcroft DW, Dosman JA, Cotton DJ. Nighttime ventilation improves respiratory failure in secondary kyphoscoliosis. *Am Rev Respir Dis* 1984;**129**:240–3.
13 Heckmatt JZ, Loh L, Dubowitz V. Night-time nasal ventilation in neuromuscular disease. *Lancet* 1990;**335**:579–82.
14 Sawicka EH, Branthwaite MA. Respiration during sleep in kyphoscoliosis. *Thorax* 1987;**42**:801–8.
15 Guilleminault C, Kurlan G, Winkle R, Miles LE. Severe kyphoscoliosis, breathing and sleep. The Quasimodo syndrome during sleep. *Chest* 1981;**79**:626–30.
16 Stradling JR, Chadwick GA, Frew AJ. Changes in ventilation and its components in normal subjects during sleep. *Thorax* 1985;**40**:364–70.
17 Douglas NJ, White DP, Pickett CK, Weil J, Zwillich CW. Respiration during sleep in normal man. *Thorax* 1982;**37**:840–4.
18 Bergofsky EH. Respiratory failure in disorders of the thoracic cage. *Am Rev Respir Dis* 1979;**119**:643–69.
19 Remmers JE. Effects of sleep on control of breathing. *Int Rev Physiol* 1981;**23**:111–47.
20 Jardim J, Farkas G, Prefant C, Thomas D, Macklem PT, Roussos C. The failing inspiratory muscles under normoxic and hypoxic conditions. *Am Rev Respir Dis* 1981;**124**:274–9.
21 Juan G, Calverley P, Talamo C, Schnader J, Roussos C. Effect of carbon dioxide on diaphragmatic function in human beings. *N Engl J Med* 1984;**310**:874–9.
22 Hudgel DW, Martin RJ, Capeheart M, Johnstone B, Hill P. Contribution of hypoventilation to sleep oxygen desaturation in chronic obstructive pulmonary disease. *J Appl Physiol* 1983;**55**:669–77.
23 Douglas NJ, Flenley DC. Breathing during sleep in patients with obstructive lung disease. *Am Rev Respir Dis* 1990;**141**:1055–70.
24 Wynne JW, Block J, Hemenway J, Hunt L, Flick MR. Disordered breathing and oxygen desaturation during sleep in patients with chronic obstructive lung disease (COPD). *Am J Med* 1979;**66**:573–9.
25 Sharp JT. The chest wall and respiratory muscles in airflow limitation. In: Roussos C, Macklem PT, eds. *The thorax.* New York: Marcel Dekker, 1985:1155–212.
26 Macklem PT. The clinical relevance of respiratory muscle research: J Burns Amberson Lecture. *Am Rev Respir Dis* 1986;**134**:812–5.
27 Sullivan CE, Berthon Jones M, Issa FG. Reversal of obstructive sleep apnoea by continuous positive airway pressure applied through the nares. *Lancet* 1983;**1**:862–5.
28 Kesten S, Rebuck AS. Nasal continuous positive airway pressure in *Pneumocystis carinii* pneumonia. *Lancet* 1988;**2**:1414–5.
29 Branson RD, Hurst JM, DeHaven CB. Mask CPAP. *Resp Care* 1985;**30**:846–57.
30 DeHaven CB, Hurst JM, Branson RD. Post extubation hypoxaemia treated with continuous positive airways pressure mask. *Crit Care Med* 1985;**13**:46–8.
31 Petrof BJ, Kimoff RJ, Levy RD, Cosio MG, Gottfried SB. Nasal continuous positive airway pressure facilitates respiratory muscle function during sleep in severe chronic obstructive pulmonary disease. *Am Rev Respir Dis* 1991;**143**:928–35.
32 Petrof BJ, Legare M, Goldberg P, Milic-Emili J, Gottfried SW. Continuous positive airway pressure reduces work of breathing and dyspnea during weaning from mechanical

NON-INVASIVE VENTILATION

ventilation in severe chronic obstructive pulmonary disease. *Am Rev Respir Dis* 1990; **141**:281–9.
33 Petrof BJ, Calderini E, Gottfried SB. Effect of CPAP on respiratory effort and dyspnea during exercise in severe COPD. *J Appl Physiol* 1990;**69**:179–88.
34 Marini JJ, Rodriguez RM, Lamb V. The inspiratory workload of patient initiated mechanical ventilation. *Am Rev Respir Dis* 1986;**134**:902–9.
35 Mayer LS, Kerby GR, Whitman RA, Shivers-Smith C. Continued evaluation of a new device for administration of continuous positive airway pressure. *Am Rev Respir Dis* 1990;**141**:A864 (Abstract).
36 Simonds AK, Cramer D, Wedzicha J. Nasal plugs (Adams circuit) for the delivery of CPAP and non-invasive intermittent positive pressure ventilation. *Thorax* 1991;**46**:291P (Abstract).
37 Branthwaite MA. Cardiorespiratory consequences of unfused idiopathic scoliosis. *Br J Dis Chest* 1986;**80**:360–9.
38 Bye PT, Ellis ER, Issa FG, Donnelly PM, Sullivan CE. Respiratory failure and sleep in neuromuscular disease. *Thorax* 1990;**45**:241–7.
39 Braun NMT, Rochester DF. Muscular weakness and respiratory failure. *Am Rev Respir Dis* 1979;**119** (suppl):123–5.
40 Simonds AK, Parker RA, Sawicka EH, Branthwaite MA. Protriptyline for nocturnal hypoventilation in restrictive chest wall disease. *Thorax* 1986;**41**:586–90.
41 Carroll N, Parker RA, Branthwaite MA. The use of protriptyline for respiratory failure in patients with chronic airflow limitation. *Eur Respir J* 1990;**3**:746–51.
42 Leger P, Robert D, Langevin B, Guez A. Chest wall deformities due to idiopathic kyphoscoliosis or sequelae of tuberculosis. *Eur Respir Rev* 1992;**2**:362–8.
43 Elliott MW, Potter N, Simonds AK. Long term follow up of patients receiving domiciliary nasal intermittent positive pressure ventilation (NIPPV) *Eur Respir J* 1993;**6**:381s (Abstract).
44 Gutierrez M, Beroiza T, Contreras G *et al.* Weekly cuirass ventilation improves blood gases and inspiratory muscle strength in patients with chronic airflow limitation and hypercarbia. *Am Rev Respir Dis* 1988;**138**:617–23.
45 Marino W. Intermittent volume cycled mechanical ventilation via nasal mask in patients with respiratory failure due to COPD. *Chest* 1991;**99**:681–4.
46 Elliott MW, Simonds AK, Carroll MP, Wedzicha JA, Branthwaite MA. Domiciliary nocturnal nasal intermittent positive pressure ventilation in hypercapnic respiratory failure due to chronic obstructive lung disease: effects on sleep and quality of life. *Thorax* 1992;**47**: 342–8.
47 Nocturnal Oxygen Therapy Trial (NOTT) group. Continuous or nocturnal oxygen therapy in hypoxaemic chronic obstructive lung disease, a clinical trial. *Ann Intern Med* 1980; **93**:391–8.
48 Medical Research Council Working Party Report. Long term domiciliary oxygen therapy in chronic hypoxic cor pulmonale complicating chronic bronchitis and emphysema. *Lancet* 1981;1:681–5.
49 Baudouin SV, Waterhouse JC, Tahtamouni T, Smith JA, Baxter J, Howard P. Long term domiciliary oxygen treatment for chronic respiratory failure reviewed. *Thorax* 1990;**45**: 195–8.
50 Walshaw MJ, Lim R, Evans CC, Hind CRK. Factors influencing compliance of patients using oxygen concentrators for long-term home oxygen therapy. *Respir Med* 1990;**84**: 331–3.
51 Burrows B, Earle RH. Course and prognosis of chronic obstructive lung disease. *N Engl J Med* 1969;**280**:397–404.
52 Sahn SA, Nett LM, Petty TL. Ten year follow-up of a comprehensive rehabilitation program for severe COPD. *Chest* 1980;77 (suppl):311–4.
53 Muir J-F. Intermittent positive pressure ventilation (IPPV) in patients with chronic obstructive pulmonary disease (COPD). *Eur Respir Rev* 1992;**2**:335–45.
54 Hodson ME, Madden BP, Steven MH, Tsang VT, Yacoub MH. Non-invasive mechanical ventilation for cystic fibrosis patients—a potential bridge to transplantation. *Eur Respir J* 1991;**4**:524–7.
55 Swami A, Evans TW, Morgan CJ, Hodson ME, Keogh BF. Conventional ventilation as a bridge to heart-lung transplantation in cystic fibrosis. *Eur Respir J* 1991;**4**:188s (Abstract).
56 Bourgeois M, Munck A, Gerardin M *et al.* Nasal ventilation in children with cystic fibrosis. *4th International Conference on Home Mechanical Ventilation* 1993:23 (Abstract).

104

57 Robert D, Gerard M, Leger P. *et al.* Domiciliary ventilation by tracheostomy for chronic respiratory failure. *Rev Fr Mal Resp* 1983;**11**:923–36.

58 Leger P, Cornette A, Bedicam JM *et al.* Long term follow-up of severe chronic respiratory insufficiency patients (n = 276) treated by home nocturnal non invasive nasal IPPV. *4th International Conference on Home Mechanical Ventilation* 1993:39 (Abstract).

59 Barois A, Estournet-Mathiaud. Ventilatory support at home in children with spinal muscular atrophies (SMA). *Eur Respir Rev* 1992;**10**:319–22.

60 Hill NS, Redline S, Carskadon M, Curran FJ, Millman RP. Sleep-disordered breathing in patients with Duchenne muscular dystrophy using negative pressure ventilators. *Chest* 1992;**102**:1656–62.

61 Braun NM, Marino WD. Effect of daily intermittent rest of respiratory muscles in patients with severe chronic airflow limitation (CAL). *Chest* 1984;**85**:59s–60s (Abstract).

62 Cropp A, Dimarco AF. Effects of intermittent negative pressure ventilation on respiratory muscle function in patients with severe chronic obstructive pulmonary disease. *Am Rev Respir Dis* 1987;**135**:1056–61.

63 Scano G, Gigliotti F, Duranti R, Spinelli A, Gorini M, Schiavina M. Changes in ventilatory muscle function with negative pressure ventilation in COPD. *Chest* 1990;**97**:322–27.

64 Gay PC, Patel AM, Viggiano RW, Hubmayr RD. Nocturnal nasal ventilation for treatment of patients with hypercapnic respiratory failure. *Mayo Clin Proc* 1991;**66**:695–703.

65 Elliott MW, Mulvey DA, Moxham J, Green M, Branthwaite MA. Domiciliary nocturnal nasal intermittent positive pressure ventilation in COPD: mechanisms underlying changes in arterial blood gas tensions. *Eur Respir J* 1991;**4**:1044–52.

66 Berthon-Jones M, Sullivan CE. Time course of change in ventilatory response to CO_2 with long-term CPAP therapy for obstructive sleep apnea. *Am Rev Respir Dis* 1987;**135**:144–7.

67 Simonds AK, Parker RA, Branthwaite MA. The effect of intermittent positive-pressure hyperinflation in restrictive chest wall disease. *Respiration* 1989;**55**:136–43.

68 McClement JH, Christianson LC, Hubayton RT, Simpson DG. The body type respirator in the treatment of chronic obstructive pulmonary disease. *Ann NY Acad Sci* 1965;**121**: 746–50.

69 Fraimow W, Cathcart RT, Goodman E. The use of intermittent positive pressure breathing in the prevention of carbon dioxide narcosis associated with oxygen therapy. *Am Rev Respir Dis* 1960;**81**:815–22.

70 Meduri GU, Conoscenti CC, Menashe P, Nair S. Noninvasive face mask ventilation in patients with acute respiratory failure. *Chest* 1989;**95**:865–70.

71 Brochard L, Isabey D, Piquet J *et al.* Reversal of acute exacerbations of chronic obstructive lung disease by inspiratory assistance with a face mask. *N Engl J Med* 1990;**323**:1523–30.

72 Elliott MW, Steven MH, Phillips GD, Branthwaite MA. Non-invasive mechanical ventilation for acute respiratory failure. *Br Med J* 1990;**300**:358–60.

73 Meduri GU, Abou-Shala N, Fox RC, Jones CB, Leeper KV, Wunderink RG. Noninvasive face mask mechanical ventilation in patients with acute hypercapnic respiratory failure. *Chest* 1991;**100**:445–54.

74 Pennock BE, Kaplan PD, Carlin BW, Sabangan JS, Magovern JA. Pressure support ventilation with a simplified ventilatory support system administered with a nasal mask in patients with respiratory failure. *Chest* 1991;**100**:1371–6.

75 Chevrolet JC, Rossi JM, Chatelain G *et al.* Intermittent mechanical ventilation as home care. *Therapeutische Umschau* 1989;**46**:697–708 (in German).

76 Foglio C, Vitacca M, Quadri A, Scalvini S, Marangoni S, Ambrosino N. Acute exacerbations in severe COLD patients. Treatment using positive pressure ventilation by nasal mask. *Chest* 1992;**101**:1533–8.

77 Benhamou D, Girault C, Faure C, Portier F, Muir JF. Nasal mask ventilation in acute respiratory failure. *Chest* 1992;**102**:912–7.

78 Bott J, Carroll MP, Conway JH *et al.* Randomised controlled trial of nasal ventilation in acute ventilatory failure due to chronic obstructive airways disease. *Lancet* 1993;**341**: 1555–7.

79 Bellon G, Mounier M, Guidicelli J, Gerard M, Alkurdi M. Nasal intermittent positive pressure ventilation in cystic fibrosis. *Eur Respir Rev* 1992;**2**:357–9.

80 Bott J, Baudouin SV, Moxham J. Nasal intermittent positive pressure ventilation in the treatment of respiratory failure in obstructive sleep apnoea. *Thorax* 1991;**46**:457–8.

81 Goldstone J, Moxham J. Weaning from mechanical ventilation. *Thorax* 1991;**46**:56–62.

82 Branthwaite MA. Getting a patient off the ventilator. *Br J Dis Chest* 1988;**8882**:16–22.

83 Goodenburger DM, Couser JI, May JJ. Successful discontinuation of ventilation via tracheostomy by substitution of nasal positive pressure ventilation. *Chest* 1992;**102**: 1277–8.

84 Udwadia ŻF, Santis GK, Steven MH, Simonds AK. Nasal ventilation to facilitate weaning in patients with chronic respiratory insufficiency. *Thorax* 1992;**47**:715–8.

85 Restrick LJ, Scott AD, Ward EM, Feneck RO, Cornwell WE, Wedzicha JA. Nasal intermittent positive-pressure ventilation in weaning intubated patients with chronic respiratory disease from assisted positive-pressure ventilation. *Resp Med* 1993;**87**:199–204.

Index

central respiratory drive 18, 67,
    82
central venous pressure 42
cerebral oedema 26
chemosensitivity 97
chest
    surgery 1, 90
    trauma 19, 36
chest wall disorders 81, 89–92,
    95, 102
    acute ventilatory failure 98, 99
    outcome of NPPV 92–3
children 34, 35, 95–7
    See also paediatric intensive care
chloral hydrate 41
chlormethiazole 22, 41
chlorpromazine 41, 50
chronic obstructive pulmonary
    disease (COPD) 18, 57, 97
    acute exacerbations 98, 99–100
    CPAP 83
    domiciliary ventilation 93–5
    doxapram 67
    negative pressure ventilation 81
    nocturnal hypoventilation 82
coma 10, 68
communication 50
continuous positive airway
    pressure (CPAP) 14, 73, 83
controlled mechanical
    ventilation 9
Copenhagen polio epidemic 1–2,
    18
cough reflex 101
cuirass 2, 80–1
cystic fibrosis 95, 98

daytime function 97–8
dextrose 47
diaphragm 64, 65, 69, 82
    pacing 81
diarrhoea 45
diazepam 40
differential ventilation 30–1
domiciliary ventilation 80
    children 95–7
    outcomes 95
    sleep 81–3
doxapram 25, 67

Draeger Evita 14
drowning 1
drug
    addiction 40
    dependency 49, 50
    withdrawal 41, 50
Duchenne muscular
    dystrophy 82, 96–7
    outcome 95
dynamic compliance 58, 67, 69
dyspnoea 26

electrolytes 48
electronic control 3, 5
emphysema
    bullous 29
    subcutaneous 22, 37, 101
encephalopathy 47
endotoxaemia 72
endotracheal intubation
    anaesthesia 21
    complications 34, 35, 38
    indications 34
    nasal 35
    tolerance 36
    tube diameter 73
    work of breathing 66
energy expenditure 46–7
energy requirements 45–6
Engstrom Erica 11, 12
ephedrine nasal drops 88
equipment failure 22
ethics 25
etomidate 7, 39
exhaustion 26
expired air resuscitation 1
extracorporeal membrane
    oxygenation 15

f/VT ratio 58–9
facial injuries 36
fat 47
feedback system 3, 5
fentanyl 40
Flow-By 13, 75
flow generators 2–3, 83, 84
fluid balance 48
flumazenil 41
fluoride 41